Secrets Of A Healer - Magic of a Reiki Master

SECRETS OF A HEALER

VOL. XI
THE REIKI MASTER'S MANUAL

Dr. Constance Santego

Maximillian Enterprises
Kelowna, BC

Secrets Of A Healer – The Reiki Master's Manual
Copyright °2024 by Dr. Constance Santego.

Copy Editor and Interior Design: Constance Santego
Book Layout: °2017 BookDesignTemplates.com
Cover Design: Jennifer Louie

Ordering Information:
Quantity sales. Special discounts are available on quantity purchases by corporations, associations, and others. For details, contact the address below.

Trade paperback ISBN: 978-1-990062-34-6

eBook ISBN 978-1-990062-35-3
Created and published In Canada. Printed and bound in the United States of America

First Edition
Published by Maximillian Enterprises
Kelowna, BC Canada
www.constancesantego.ca

Dedication

To all my Reiki instructors and all other instructors and practitioners who practice this marvelous hands-on healing technique.

*"Your hands hold the power
to heal."*

—Dr. Constance Santego

ALSO BY DR. CONSTANCE SANTEGO

FICTION
The Nine Spiritual Gifts Series: *(based on actual events)*
Journey of a Soul – (Vol 1 Michael)
Language of a Soul – (Vol 2 Gabriel)
Prophecy of a Soul – (Vol 3 Bath Kol)
Healing of a Soul – (Vol 4 Raphael)
Miracles of a Soul – (Vol 5 Hamied)
Knowledge of a Soul – (Vol 6 Raziel)

NONFICTION
The Intuitive Life, The Gift of Prophecy, Third Edition
Fairy Tales, Dreams and Reality… Where Are You On Your Path? Second Edition
Your Persona… The Mask You Wear
Angelic Lifestyle, A Vibrant Lifestyle
Angelic Lifestyle 42-Day Energy Cleanse
Archangel Michael's Soul Retrieval Guide
Tesla and the Future of Energy Medicine
Scaling Beyond 6 Figures: *Strategies for Health & Wellness Professionals*
Beyond the Mind: *Harnessing the Power of Astral Projection for Creative Awakening*
Bend, Don't Break: *Finding Your Way Back to Abundance*

SECRETS OF A HEALER, SERIES:
Magic Of Aromatherapy (Vol I)
Magic Of Reflexology (Vol II)
Magic Of The Gifts (Vol III)
Magic Of Muscle Testing (Vol IV)
Magic Of Iridology (Vol V)
Magic Of Massage (Vol VI)
Magic Of Hypnotherapy (Vol VII)
Magic Of Reiki (Vol VIII)
Magic Of Advanced Aromatherapy (Vol IX)
Magic Of Esthetics (Vol X)

ADULT COLORING JOURNALS
SERIES - ZEN COLORING:
Quantum Energy and Mindful Living Journal (Vol 1)
Reiki Energy Journal (Vol 2)
Nine Spiritual Gifts Journal (Vol 3)
I Forgive Journal (Vol 4)

SERIES – COLORING PROSPERITY:
Genie-Inspired Mandalas and Wealth Journal (Vol 1)
Entrepreneurial Mindset Reboot (Vol 2)

FOR CHILDREN
I am Big Tonight. I Don't Need the Light!

COOKBOOK
My Favorite Recipes, with a Hint of Giggle

Contents

Preface...xiv

Note to Reader...xvi

Learning Outcome xviii

REIKI LEVEL I THE APPRENTICE 1

    Reiki Level 1 Lesson Plan 2

    Dr. Usui 3

Three Levels of Reiki.. 5

What is Reiki? 8

    Reiki = Life-Force Energy 9

Origin - How Did Dr. Usui Learn The Knowledge...................... 10

The Four Miracles.. 11

Just For Today 13

Dr. Constance's Lineage 14

How Energy Works 15

Understanding Chakras: The Basics..................................... 17

Kidney Breathing And The Hui Yin.. 23

Water Ritual.. 24

LEVEL 1 MEDITATION FOR ATTUNEMENT............................ 27

    Part "One" Of Level 1 Attunement Meditation.............. 27

    Level 1 Reiki Symbols 33

    Part "Two" Of Level 1 Attunement Meditation.............. 42

Reiki 21-Day Cleanse.. 45

Reiki Self-Treatment Hand Positions.................................... 48

    Reiki Self-Treatment 49

Reiki Breathing Exercise:..50

Quick Energizer: 51

Sleep Help:..51

Reiki Self Treatment - Full Body..52

Reiki Level 1 – Apprentice Homework.......................................55

REIKI LEVEL 2 – THE PRACTITIONER......................................57

Reiki Level 2 Lesson Plan 58

Second Degree Reiki 59

LEVEL 2 MEDITATION FOR ATTUNEMENT............................61

Part "One" Of Level 2 Attunement Meditation 61

Reiki Level 2 Symbols..66

Part "Two" Of Level 2 Attunement Meditation 85

A Reiki Treatment On A Client...88

Distant Healing 95

Distant Healing Visualization:..96

Full Body Absentee Treatment..97

The Hand Sandwich Treatment..98

Reiki Practitioner's Mind and Personal Issues During Mental or
Emotional Reiki Sessions...99

Mental Healing 104

Emotional Healing 109

Reiki In Daily Life..112

Reiki Level 2 – Practitioner Homework...................................114

Reiki Level 2 – Client Case Study Example.............................115

Opening Your Own Reiki Clinic: The Basics............................117

If Not Charging Any Money 117

If Charging Money 117

REIKI LEVEL 3 – MASTER 121

   Reiki Level 3 Lesson Plan......................................122

   Reiki Spiritual Healing...123

LEVEL 3 MEDITATION FOR ATTUNEMENT 126

   Part "One" Of Level 3 Attunement Meditation 126

   Reiki "Master" Symbols..134

   Raku Affirmation 139

   Part "Two" Of Level 3 Attunement Meditation 152

Understanding Auras 155

   Essential Knowledge for Reiki Level 3 Students...........155

Advanced Reiki Practices for Level 3 Students 159

   Chakra Clearing 160

   Harmonizing Chakras..164

   Grounding Exercise 165

   Causal Plane Work 166

Reiki Master = Teacher 170

   Teaching Reiki Level 3: Master Level and the Ability to
Teach and Initiate 170

Preparing to Teach Reiki 175

   Teaching Reiki Level 1: The Foundation......................176

   Teaching Reiki Level 2: Deepening the Connection........178

   Teaching Reiki Level 3: Master Level 180

Teaching Guidelines for Reiki Level 3 Students 182

   Advertising Your Classes.......................................182

   Preparing Materials..183

   Conducting Your Classes..183

Attunement Procedure for Each Reiki Level 186

Reiki Certificates Examples..189
Companion Books...195
Bibliography...198
Message From The Author 208

Preface

The Miracle of Reiki

In 1999, Reiki was one of the first modalities taught at my new school. Before my Reiki Master, Nefertiti, came and offered Level I & II courses, I had no idea what Reiki was. That amazing weekend course profoundly changed my life.

At that time, practices like Reiki were often dismissed as "woo, woo" or hocus pocus. Many people even believed Reiki to be the Devil's work simply because they couldn't understand or perceive its benefits. It's strange how quickly society labels something as evil when it is unfamiliar. For example, marijuana was once considered bad, but now it's recognized for its medicinal properties, particularly for pain relief in cancer patients.

I'm incredibly happy and grateful that society changed its Reiki perspective. It's wonderful to see it being accepted and appreciated for the positive impact it can have, especially now that it is being offered in cancer clinics.

Note to Reader

Reiki is not intended to replace traditional medical techniques. Persons with physical, mental, emotional, and spiritual problems should seek the service of a professional psychologist or Doctor.

Your Doctor still plays a vital role in your health care. For example, if you break my leg, You will need a Doctor, all the nurses, and staff in the Hospital.

Integrated Medicine focuses on "**our**" significant role in caring for our health. What we put into our bodies, how hard we work our bodies, the stress level we allow into our everyday lives, and the positive or negative energy we attract around us all play a role in our well-being.

Reiki is an excellent technique for relaxation, stress relief, clearing the mind, improving self-awareness, self-empowerment, and possibly a miracle. However, you are ALWAYS in control of your health, and Reiki cannot heal you alone. Only you can do that.

A legal *(Signed by your Reiki Master)* Reiki Level 2 certificate is required if you are to "charge $" to "treat" others, and a Reiki Level 3 certificate is required if you are to "charge $" and "teach" others!

Learning Outcome

This book is a comprehensive Reiki Master's manual, providing detailed information for each Reiki level: I, II, and III. It is designed to guide both new and experienced practitioners through the essential components of Reiki training and practice. By the end of this manual, readers will have a thorough understanding of the following:

- **Level 1- Shoden/Apprentice**:
  - Introduction to Reiki, its history, and principles.
  - Basic hand positions for self-healing and healing others.
  - Techniques for clearing and balancing the chakras.
- **Level 2 – Okuden/Practitioner**:
  - Advanced healing techniques, including mental and emotional healing.
  - Introduction and usage of Reiki symbols such as Cho Ku Rei, Sei He Ki, and Hon Sha Ze Sho Nen.
  - Methods for distant healing and sending Reiki across time and space.
- **Level 3 – Shinpiden/Master**:
  - Master-level teachings, including the use of the Dai Ko Myo symbol.

- Instructions on how to perform attunements and teach Reiki to others.
- Advanced practices for spiritual growth and connection to higher consciousness.

- **Symbols:**
  - Detailed explanations and applications of all Reiki symbols used in each level.
  - Step-by-step guides on how to draw and invoke the symbols during healing sessions.

- **Hands-on Healing Techniques:**
  - Practical techniques for performing hands-on Reiki sessions.
  - Guidelines for harmonizing and balancing chakras through touch.
  - Methods for grounding and protecting oneself and others during healing.

This manual is intended to be a complete resource for Reiki practitioners, providing all the necessary tools and knowledge to become a confident and skilled Reiki Master. Whether you are beginning your journey with Level 1 or advancing to Level 3, this book will support your growth and development in the practice of Reiki.

REIKI LEVEL I
THE APPRENTICE

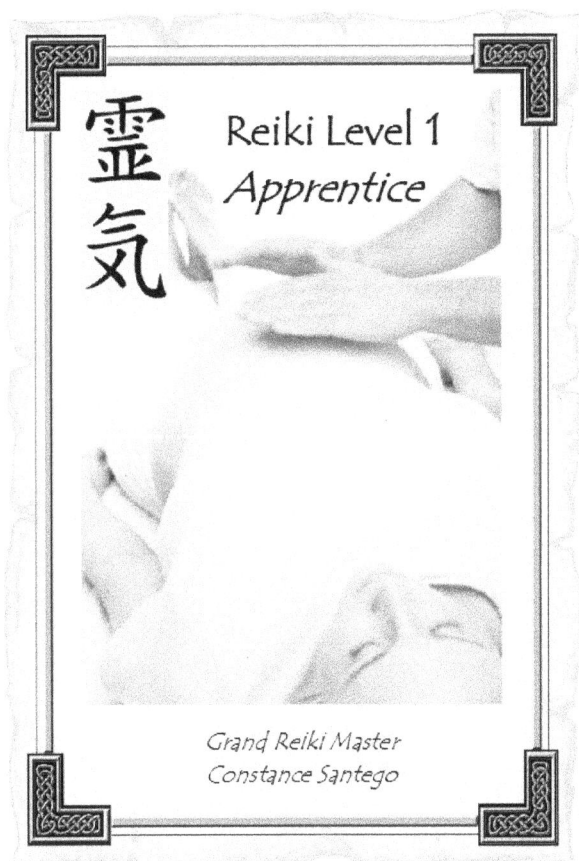

Reiki Level 1
Apprentice

Grand Reiki Master
Constance Santego

Level 1: Shoden

Shoden, meaning "First Teaching" or "Beginning Transmission," is the introductory level of Reiki training. It focuses on the basics of Reiki, including its history, principles, and fundamental techniques.

Reiki Level 1 Lesson Plan

3-hour live class

1st part of the class
Go through these pages:

- Dr. Usui
- Three levels of Reiki
  - Physical
  - Mental / Emotional
  - Spiritual
- What is Reiki
- Origin: How did Dr Usui learn the knowledge
- Four miracles
- Just for today
- Lineage (do mine and yours)
- How energy works (Is in Secrets of a Healer – Magic of Reiki)
- Chakras (In Secrets of a Healer – Magic of Reiki)
- Break for 15 min

2nd part of the class
- *Listen and Subscribe*
  https://youtu.be/dPmM6Zuua5Q
or *Read* the "Apprentice" Meditation
  - Draw the level 1 symbol on each student
  - Finish meditation (this is where they meet "their" Reiki Master)
- Have each student talk about what they experienced

3rd part of the class
- Practice each hand position.

Dr. Usui

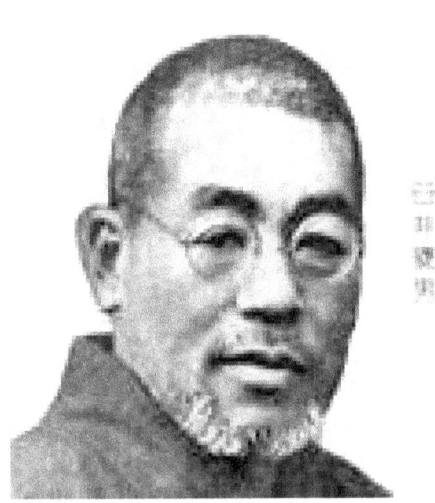

Reiki originated in Tibet and was discovered in the nineteenth century by a Japanese monk, Dr. Mikao Usui, born to a wealthy Buddhist family (15 August 1865 – 9 March 1926).

Dr. Usui's family was able to give their son a well-rounded education for the time. As a child, Dr. Usui studied in a Buddhist monastery where he was taught martial arts, swordsmanship, and the Japanese form of Chi Kung, known as Kiko (Qigong).

Adding to his comprehension of Japanese, Dr. Usui learned Sanskrit and Chinese, as well as other languages, so that he could study each manuscript himself, and nothing would be 'lost' or 'misinterpreted' in translation.

In the mid-1800s, Dr. Mikao Usui studied ancient Sanskrit writings and Jesus' healing technique. Dr. Usui was transfixed in unraveling the secrets of healing. So, he went on a quest to find out how Buddha and Jesus had healed with their hands.

He found what he thought would be essential to physical healing in the Sanskrit sutras. He discovered symbols, formulas, and intellectual writings but did not find the method or technique.

He asked for advice on what to do from the Abbott of the Zen Buddhist monastery where he was staying. They decided that he should go to the scared Mount Kurama, outside of Kyoto in the Kuriyama district, which is situated in the central region of Hokkaido. The name *Kuriyama means 'Chestnut Mountain' in Japanese.*

Three Levels of Reiki

- ➢ 1st Degree/Level 1 – Shoden/Apprentice
  - o Physical Self-healing,
- ➢ 2nd Degree/Level 2 – Okuden/Practitioner
  - o Healing others,
  - o Physical, Mental, and Emotional healing,
- ➢ 3rd Degree/Level 3 – Shinpiden/Master/Teacher
  - o Teaching others.
  - o Spiritual healing.

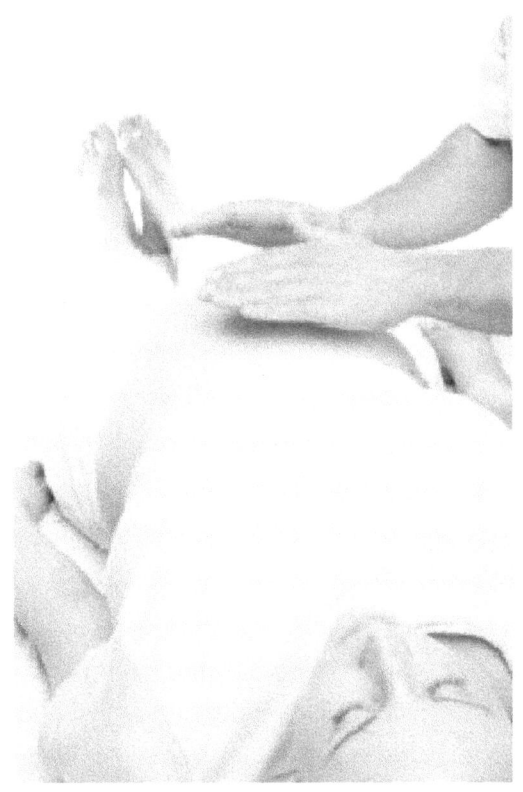

FIRST-DEGREE REIKI, LEVEL I – SHODEN/APPRENTICE

Body – All about self-healing!

WHAT DO YOU LEARN?
- 1st degree Reiki Attunement (Meet your Reiki Master in Spirit),
- Reiki Energy,
- Chakras,
- Physical Healing,
- Self-Healing using the seven major Chakras and the 16 minor Chakra hand positions.

SECOND-DEGREE REIKI, LEVEL II – OKUDEN/PRACTITIONER

Body & Mind – All about healing ANOTHER person!

WHAT DO YOU LEARN NEW?
- 2nd degree Reiki Attunement,
- Using the hand position of level 1 (7 major Chakras and the 16 minor Chakras) and combining it with 361 Tsubo points on the body,
- Chakra Crystal Healing,
- Chakra Pendulum Healing,
- Mental & Emotional Healing,
- Distance Healing.

THIRD-DEGREE REIKI, LEVEL III – SHINPIDEN/MASTER

Body, Mind & Soul - All about TEACHING another person!

WHAT DO YOU LEARN NEW?
- 3rd degree Reiki Attunement,
- You learned physical healing in Level 1, mental & emotional healing in Level 2, and now, in Level 3, you will learn Spiritual Healing,
- PLUS!!! How to teach Reiki to others. You become the Teacher!

The degree of Reiki does not equate to the amount of energy you have to use. The degree only refers to the knowledge you learn within each level.

What is Reiki?

Reiki is a hands-on-healing energy technique used on the body's chakras and tsubus (meridian points).

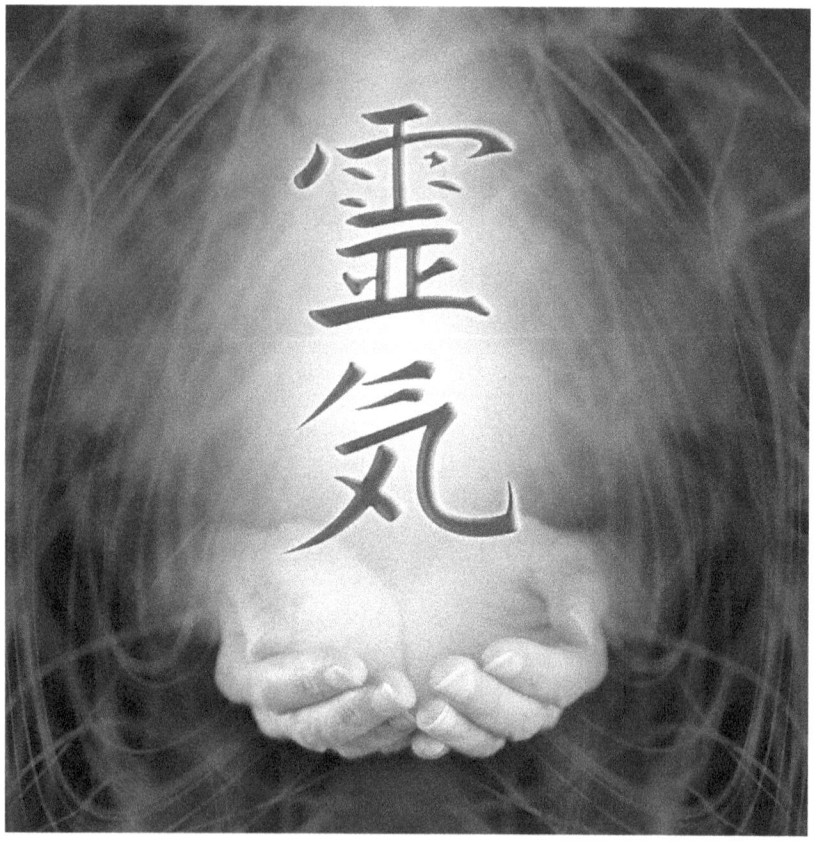

Reiki = Life-Force Energy

Reiki is one of the most ancient healing methods known to mankind. It is used as an alternative therapy for treating physical, emotional, mental, and spiritual dis-ease.

Reiki is the Japanese word for 'Universal Life-force Energy.' The definition of 'Rei' is a universal, mysterious power, transcendental spirit. 'Ki' is described as the vital life-force energy. Together, they could mean 'Spirit Energy' or 'Power Energy.' However, the essence is more that of 'Universal Life-force Energy – All-Encompassing.'

The tradition of Reiki is referred to in the 3500-year-old writings in Sanskrit, where writing was used as a means of communication and dialogue by the Hindu Celestial Gods and was termed as Deva-Vani ('Deva' Gods - 'Vani' language) as it was believed to have been generated by the God Brahma who passed it to the Rishis (sages) living in celestial bodies, who then communicated the same to their earthly disciples from where it spread on earth. Today, it is used by the Indo-Aryans (the ancient language of Hinduism), and it is also widely used in Jainism, Buddhism, and Sikhism.

Reiki is not a religion or belief system – it holds no doctrine. It is a healing modality that combines the power of God's life-force healing energy and your body's Chakra system.

Origin –
How Did Dr. Usui Learn The Knowledge

For 21 days, he would fast and meditate to see if he could gain insight into the use of the information that he found. Dr. Usui collected 21 stones to keep track of his time in a cave on the mountain. Each day, he threw one stone away and then meditated and fasted.

On the morning of the 21st day, he still had not received the knowledge he sought. As he prayed that morning that before dawn, he would be shown the light and how to use the 'keys to healing' that he had found in the scriptures, he threw away his last stone.

Disappointed that evening for not accomplishing his quest, he stood up to leave, and as he did so, a little beam of light way off on the horizon started to move toward him. As it came closer, it became bigger and bigger, nearly frightening him to death. He had spent years on this quest and was not about to run now. Finally, as he braced himself, the light struck him in the middle of his forehead and knocked him out.

In his dream state, he experienced a rainbow of colors, and the Sanskrit symbols, their use, and meanings were drawn in the sky. In his initial attunement, Dr. Usui received all the keys to healing. He vowed never to forget them or allow them to be lost.

The Four Miracles

Dr. Usui was ecstatic about his experience and newfound knowledge and quickly started down the mountain back to Kyoto and the monastery. On his journey back, the 'Four Miracles of Reiki' happened.

Miracle number one, in his haste, he tripped and stubbed his toe. He instinctively bent down, held his aching toe between his hands, and soon realized that the pain and bleeding had stopped. He also noticed a great deal of heat-generating out of his hands.

Miracle number two happened when he broke his twenty-one-day fast by ordering a full meal at a home that served travelers. He ate the entire meal and did not suffer any indigestion or discomfort.

Miracle number three, the young girl serving him, suffered from an abscessed tooth. Again, Dr. Usui placed his hands on the swelling, and within moments, the pain and swelling disappeared.

Miracle number four happened back at the monastery. The Abbott was in dire pain from an arthritis attack. Dr. Usui placed his hands on the area of pain while sharing his experiences with the Abbott; very quickly, the pain disappeared.

After much meditation and consulting with the Abbott, Dr. Usui decided to use his new healing knowledge, which he called Reiki, on the poor, diseased, and crippled. So for many years, he worked with these people, giving healing.

But years later, one day, he noticed that many of the people he healed had returned to their lives as beggars. When he asked why, they replied that it was much easier, with no responsibilities.

Frustrated with this and feeling like he had failed, Dr. Usui realized that even though he had healed, he did not teach any responsibility. Therefore, an equal energy exchange, monetary or other, was required from that day forward.

In 1922, Dr. Usui *(Usui Sensei -teacher or instructor)* founded his first Reiki clinic and school in Tokyo and taught Reiki. He trained approximately sixteen Reiki Masters. Before his death, he gave Dr. Chujiro Hayashi the responsibility of preserving and passing on the tradition of Reiki.

It was Dr. Hayashi who developed the three levels of Reiki.

As World War II was coming, Dr. Hayashi feared Reiki's survival, knowing that many men would die in the war. So Dr. Hayashi decided to train a Japanese woman living in Hawaii, Mrs. Hawayo Takata.

Mrs. Takata brought Reiki training to the United States and Canada and was the one who decided to charge a fee for each level of training.

Just For Today

Dr. Usui created the 'Five Principles of Reiki.'

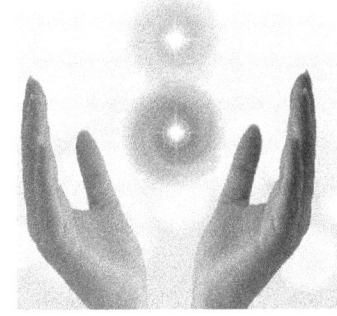

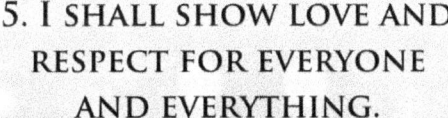

JUST FOR TODAY,

1. I WILL NOT WORRY,

2. I SHALL DO MY WORK HONESTLY,

3. I SHALL ACCEPT MY MANY BLESSINGS,

4. I SHALL DEAL WITH ANGER APPROPRIATELY,

5. I SHALL SHOW LOVE AND RESPECT FOR EVERYONE AND EVERYTHING.

Dr. Constance's Lineage

I was initiated into Reiki Level 1 & 2 in September 1999, by an American lady who called herself Nefertiti.

I received my Reiki Master from Margaret back in 2000.

Lineage

In 2023, I received my Doctorate and Ph.D. in Natural Medicine. In 2017, my name was changed to Constance Santego. In the year 2010, I, Connie Brummet, was attuned to Grand Reiki Mastery by Spirit, and in 2000, I was attuned to Reiki Mastery by Margaret Ripple, who was attuned in 1998 by Wendy Koenig, who was attuned in 1997 by Laurie Grant.

In 1989, Laurie Grant was attuned by James Davis, who Dr. Arthur Robertson attuned. Dr. Robertson was initiated in the 1970s into the Reiki system by Master teacher Virginia.

Samdahl was the first Occidental Reiki Master initiated by Hawayo Takata.

In the late 1970s and early 1980s, Dr. Robertson studied and shared with Reiki Master Teacher Iris Ishikuro, who also was initiated into the system by Mrs. Takata.

1938, Mrs. Takata received her Master's attunement from Mr. Chujiro Hayashi. Mr. Hayashi received his Reiki Mastership from Dr. Usui in 1925. Dr. Usui received his attunement from Spirit in 1922.

How Energy Works

Reiki energy heals the person by flowing through the affected parts of the vital or auric field (aura) and balancing the area. Each person has a field that surrounds their physical body. During a Reiki session, the cosmic energy balances the person's vibratory rate and frequency of their vital field (aura).

Imagine, if you like, that the vital field (aura) is like a pool of water. The water can be polluted by adding toxins, such as chemicals, mud, or objects. The water can also become stale if it is not fed fresh oxygen or has any movement. After some time, green or blue algae can grow, and the water becomes rancid, killing anything that enters.

Water is a known conductor; the clearer the water, the better its conductive ability. So even though your vital field (aura) is not liquid like water and is invisible to most people's naked eye, it radiates the clarity of your body, mind, and soul's pool of health.

During a Reiki session, the intent of the life-force energy coming down from the Cosmos is channeled through the person's crown, brow, throat, and heart chakras, then is channeled through their hands to the chakra and tsubo area(s) that need balancing.

When a person is attuned to 2nd and 3rd Degree Reiki, this energy heals and balances the emotional, mental, and spiritual bodies of the person and their physical body.

Additional Context and Benefits:

Reiki is not only a method of energy healing but also a way to promote relaxation and reduce stress. Practitioners believe that by channeling positive energy into the body, Reiki helps to enhance the body's natural healing processes. This practice can also complement other medical or therapeutic techniques to relieve side effects and promote recovery.

During a session, the practitioner may use various hand positions and either lightly touch the body or hover their hands just above it. Sessions typically last 30 to 60 minutes, depending on the individual's needs and the practitioner's approach.

Many people who receive Reiki report experiencing a sense of deep relaxation, warmth, and well-being. While scientific research on Reiki is still developing, many practitioners and recipients believe in its effectiveness based on personal experiences and historical usage.

Reiki is also accessible to anyone who wishes to learn it. With proper attunement and training, individuals can practice self-Reiki or offer healing to others, fostering a sense of community and shared wellness.

More is taught on this subject matter in my book,
"Secrets of a Healer – Magic of Reiki (Vol X)

Trade paperback ISBN: 978-1-7772220-0-0
eBook ISBN 978-1-7772220-1-7

Understanding Chakras: The Basics

What are Chakras?

Chakras are energy centers within the human body that are believed to regulate various physical, emotional, and spiritual functions. The word "chakra" comes from the Sanskrit word for "wheel" or "disk," indicating that these energy centers are like spinning wheels of energy located along the spine.

How Many Chakras Are There?

While some traditions mention various numbers of chakras, the most commonly referenced system identifies seven primary chakras, each located at a specific point along the spine, from the base to the crown of the head. These seven chakras are:

Root Chakra (Muladhara)

Location: Base of the spine

Color: Red

Element: Earth

Associated with: Basic survival needs, grounding, stability, and security.

Imbalances may cause: Anxiety, fears, and physical issues with the legs, feet, and lower back.

Sacral Chakra (Svadhisthana)

Location: Lower abdomen, about two inches below the navel

Color: Orange

Element: Water

Associated with: Emotions, creativity, sexuality, and pleasure.

Imbalances may cause: Emotional instability, sexual dysfunction, and issues with the reproductive organs and kidneys.

Solar Plexus Chakra (Manipura)

Location: Upper abdomen, around the stomach area

Color: Yellow

Element: Fire

Associated with: Personal power, self-esteem, and confidence.

Imbalances may cause: Digestive issues, low self-esteem, and lack of self-control.

Heart Chakra (Anahata)

Location: Center of the chest, just above the heart

Color: Green

Element: Air

Associated with: Love, compassion, and relationships.

Imbalances may cause: Heart and lung issues, emotional distress, and difficulties in relationships.

Throat Chakra (Vishuddha)

Location: Throat

Color: Blue

Element: Ether (Space)

Associated with: Communication, self-expression, and truth.

Imbalances may cause: Throat and neck problems, communication issues, and difficulty expressing oneself.

Third Eye Chakra (Ajna)

Location: Forehead, between the eyebrows

Color: Indigo

Element: Light

Associated with: Intuition, insight, and psychic abilities.

Imbalances may cause: Headaches, vision problems, and difficulty concentrating.

Crown Chakra (Sahasrara)

Location: Top of the head

Color: Violet or white

Element: Thought

Associated with: Spiritual connection, enlightenment, and higher consciousness.

Imbalances may cause: Spiritual disconnection, confusion, and neurological issues.

How Do Chakras Work?

Chakras are believed to receive, process, and transmit energy throughout the body. When they are open and balanced, energy flows freely, promoting physical, emotional, and spiritual well-being. However, if a chakra becomes blocked or unbalanced, it can lead to various physical and emotional issues.

Balancing the Chakras

There are many ways to balance and align the chakras, including:

- **Meditation:** Focusing on each chakra and visualizing its associated color and location can help balance the energy centers.
- **Yoga:** Specific poses and practices can target and open different chakras.
- **Reiki and Energy Healing:** Practitioners use techniques to channel energy and clear blockages in the chakras.
- **Crystals:** Certain crystals are associated with each chakra and can be used in healing practices.
- **Affirmations:** Positive statements related to the qualities of each chakra can help promote balance.
- **Aromatherapy:** Essential oils corresponding to each chakra can be used to enhance healing practices.

Understanding and working with chakras can be a powerful tool for achieving holistic health and well-being. Paying attention to these energy centers and ensuring they are balanced can enhance your physical health, emotional stability, and spiritual growth.

More is taught on this subject matter in my book,
"Secrets of a Healer – Magic of Reiki (Vol X)

Trade paperback ISBN: 978-1-7772220-0-0
eBook ISBN 978-1-7772220-1-7

Kidney Breathing And The Hui Yin

When you attune students, it is necessary for you, the teacher, and ideally for your students to direct the RAKU fire energy up the spine and into the pineal gland. This re-energizes the entire body and raises spiritual consciousness. Do the following three steps:

1) **Do Kidney Breathing:** Place the palm of your hands on your lower back over your kidneys. Direct your breath into the kidneys, expanding them. Your hands should rise with every inhalation and lie flat at the end of every exhalation. This type of breathing will increase your RAKU energy if you practice this every day.

2) **Contact Your Hui Yin:** The Hui Yin is an acupressure point between your anus and genitals. Breath normally again while feeling like you are pulling this point up into your body as you contract it (women may be familiar with the term "Kegel Exercise"). This step directs the RAKU fire energy up along the spinal column.

3) **Combine the Two: First, contract your Hui Yin, then take a Kidney Breath through your nose, imagining a mist of energy going down to the base of your spine along with your breath.** The mist intake swirls around the base of your spine and then moves up it as if it were in a hollow tube, entering and swirling in your head. Now, release the mist through your mouth with a hissing sound, and make this sound by placing your tongue at the ridge behind your front teeth. Make an "F" sound as you drop your tongue, making a "St"

sound as you release your breath and drop your Hui Yin.

Note: During the attunements, you, as the teacher, should hold your Hui Yin until you've released your Kidney Breath with your last student.

KIDNEY BREATH

1) TEACHER: OPEN THE STUDENT'S PALMS
2) STUDENT: HOLD HUI YIN
3) TEACHER: DRAW APPROPRIATE SYMBOLS
4) STUDENT: MAKE AN "F" SOUND AS THEY DROP THEIR TONGUE, MAKING A "ST" SOUND AS THEY RELEASE THEIR BREATH AND DROP THEIR HUI YIN.

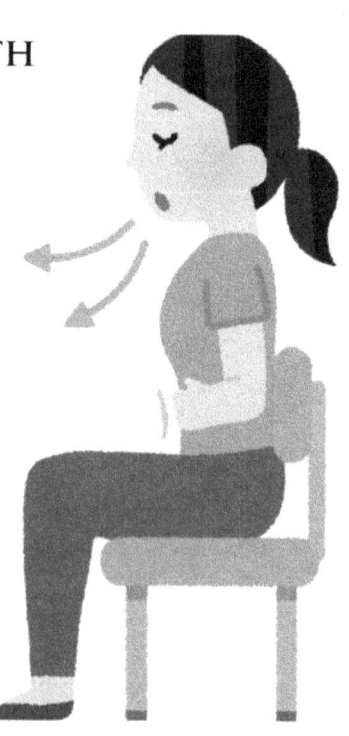

Water Ritual

Water purifies, conducts electricity, and amplifies the effectiveness of the symbols one is attuned to.

Prepare The Water:

1) Get centered.
2) Call upon your Reiki Master In Spirit and Higher Self to assist you in attuning the water.
3) Squeeze about half a teaspoon of fresh lemon juice into a clear glass or plastic cup. (One per student)
4) Fill each glass half full with distilled water.
    - For 1" Degree, draw a RAKU and CHOKUREI symbol over each glass.
    - For 2" Degree, draw a RAKU and SEIHEKI symbol over each glass. For 1" & 2" combined, draw all three symbols over each glass.
    - For the Master's Degree, draw a RAKU symbol over each glass.
5) Have the student hold the glass in prayer form over their Solar Plexus, palms on each side with fingers touching.
6) Say to students:
    a. "Pull up your Hui Yin and take a Kidney Breath, visualizing, knowing, or feeling the mist of energy going down to the base of your spine. Follow it as it swirls around your spine's base, then moves up the spine as if it were in a hollow tube, entering and swirling in your head. Exhale your breath through your mouth, making a hissing sound. While exhaling,

imagine the mist of energy passing into your glass and releasing your Hui Yin. Draw the attuning symbol horizontally over your glass".

b. Have the students say the following:

"I exercise the O SUI CHING (spirit of water) to receive the Divine Benediction of Fire. I declare this to be true, so in the name of the Holy of Holies, so be it."

c. Now, have the students draw the appropriate attuning symbol over their glass and drink the water.

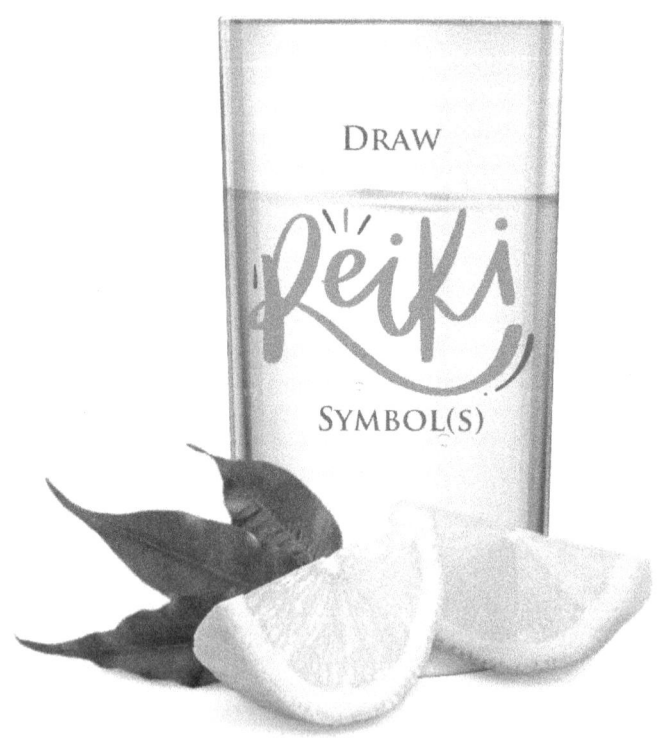

LEVEL 1 MEDITATION FOR ATTUNEMENT

You have a choice:

1) Listen to the meditation on YouTube
   https://youtu.be/dPmM6Zuua5Q

Or

2) In class:
   a. Read the 1st part of the meditation,
   b. Draw the reiki symbols on each student's crown, heart chakras, and both palms. *(by holding Hui Yin and taking a Kidney Breath),*
   c. Read 2nd part of the meditation,
   d. Water Ritual (Draw the Symbols over the lemon water),
   e. Say the Raku Kei Affirmation

Part "One" Of Level 1 Attunement Meditation

Meeting Your Reiki Master

Your Reiki Master in Spirit

Everyone is granted a special companion whose job is to help you facilitate a Reiki session. Your Reiki Master will be shown to you in your attunement to the Reiki energy. This is a very special experience; some feel wonderful tingles, see beautiful colors and images, hear music, and just know it to be true.

You will meet your Reiki Master through a meditation that will be read to you by your Reiki Master/Instructor – in class or on YouTube online. Everyone seems to get someone or something a little different. It will always come to you in the form that you can handle. I have had students who get a person —male or female, old or young, some an animal, some a color, some just a name, and some are so scared they don't seem to get anything. Just relax...and enjoy the meditation.

A State of Relaxation

This relaxation technique is done at the beginning of each attunement. Realize that this is not the only relaxation meditation you can use. I use this one because it creates a hypnotic state that allows you to attune your students at both the conscious and unconscious levels. It is important, as you proceed with this relaxation that a pause of about 5 seconds long occurs between each statement.

Read this Meditation:

"Close your eyes....get comfortable.....get really relaxed..... Take a deep breath all the way down to the bottom of your lungs...Now, let your breath out slowly and completely...Concentrate your attention behind your eyes....relax all the muscles in your eyes..... Relax them completely... Relax them so much that they just won't open....And now that they are relaxed test them.....If they are relaxed, they just won't open.....Good.....Now take another deep breath... Feel it as is expands every part of your lungs.....Now exhale slowly and completely....Let that same relaxation in your eye muscles go all the way down to your toes.....Let go completely. Use your imagination.....Now get ready to go beyond yourself....From this point on, let all outside noises increase your awareness on my voice....Let my voice be your voice....Relax your toes completely....Concentrate all your attention in your feet. Let go....All the muscles in your legs....concentrate on relaxing them now..... Your lower legs... and your upper legs....Now concentrate on relaxing your hips....your lower abdomen....and your stomach....Relax your lower back....Relax your chest....and your upper back....Not falling asleep.... Still very much aware of everything that is going on....Able to hear my voice clearly....Now relax all of the muscles in your shoulders and neck....Relax your arms....all the way down to your finger tips....Now concentrate on relaxing your jaw... Relax it freely....Relax your tongue....Now relax all of the muscles in your face....your mouth....your eyes....your jaw....and your forehead.... You're very deeply relaxed now....Not out of touch with reality. Very much in tune with everything I am saying. Completely aware of your surroundings....just very, very deeply relaxed....Now, you have reached a level of deep physical relaxation.

Let's concentrate on deep mental relaxation....For mental relaxation, I will count slowly from 100 to 98, so that you may double your relaxation with each number. When you reach 98, just let the number vanish. Here we go....100....Now double your relaxation, just let go....99....double again your relaxation, now even more relaxed....98....double one more time your relaxation....Now let the numbers vanish....Let them disappear.... This is a nice stage of relaxation. Not out of touch with reality....deeply in tune with everything I am saying....Completely aware of your surroundings....just very intent upon my voice....Allowing all noises to increase your attention....Repeat mentally the following affirmation:

In the province of the mind, I am unlimited.

(Repeat 6 more times)

The next time you go into meditation, you will go even deeper....It will work even better....faster....deeper.

Now, you will move to the higher side of yourself....Pure spirit....A being of light.... You are not your body. Concentrate your attention in your toes. Notice you have toes...and they are relaxed....but you are not your toes....Notice your feet now....and your lower legs....and your upper legs.... You are not these either....As you relax more and more, concentrate your attention on my voice....Notice you have hips, but you are not your hips....Notice your stomach....your chest....and your breathing....going in and out. You are not your stomach....and you are not your chest....and you are not your breathing. Notice your entire back....that's not who you are either. Notice your shoulders.... You're aware that they're there....they're yours....But you are not your shoulders....and you are not your arms either. Notice you have a neck....But you are not your neck.... Switch your consciousness to your jaw now....You are not your jaw. You are not your tongue....nor are you all the muscles in your face........including your nose....your eyes..........and your mouth.... You are not those....Notice your thoughts now....and you have thoughts....but you are not your thoughts....Go even deeper now....Give me your full attention....Concentrate on my voice.

It is now time to raise your vibrational rate with feelings of love and strong positive thoughts. You may do this by surrounding yourself with a beautiful protective white light. This white light represents truth....forgiveness....your ideal concept of the Source, and all that is good. Picture this white light now starting to glow in your heart.

Allow this white light to glow within your heart....Let it increase. Feel its warmth and purity. Allow it to extend and to radiate out of your heart so that it envelops your body....Completely surrounding you in a cocoon of pure, vibrant white light.... This white light is the Source's perfect presence. You may actually see it....feel it....or sense it....but all you really have to do is to know it to be there. It will always be with you. You now have the protective white light around you so that your subconscious mind is only open to suggestions that are helpful and beneficial to you.....Bathe yourself in the white light....Notice that you are light.... You are pure spirit....A dearly beloved child of the Source....Beyond time and space. Feel your light extending....Emanate your light into infinity....

You are pure light....unconditional pure love....pure compassion....pure forgiveness. You are beyond the beyond....you are one with the universe.

Attune the Student:

1) *While the student holds their "Hui Yin," open their crown chakra with the Raku Symbol, then draw the Reiki Level 1 - Chokurei symbol into their crown, heart, and palms.*
2) *Now, the student takes a "Kidney Breath."*
3) *Close their crown with the Raku symbol...*
4) *Then, continue the second part of the meditation...*

Level 1 Reiki Symbols

Using Reiki Symbols: Saying, Thinking, Seeing, and Drawing

Reiki symbols like Chokurei are powerful tools in energy healing, and there are multiple ways to use them during a session. Any of these ways can evoke the Reiki symbol and its energy. Here's how a person can say, think, see, or draw these symbols effectively:

1. Saying the Symbols

Chokurei (Show Ku Ray):

- Verbal Invocation: Say "Chokurei" out loud to activate its power. You can repeat it several times to enhance the energy.
- Affirmation: Use phrases like "I invoke the power of Chokurei for healing" or "Chokurei, please amplify the Reiki energy."

2. Thinking the Symbols

Chokurei:

- Mental Visualization: Picture the Chokurei symbol in your mind's eye. Imagine drawing it mentally, starting from the top and creating the spiral.
- Focus: Concentrate on the symbol and its purpose, visualizing it channeling energy into the area of need.

3. Seeing the Symbols

Chokurei:

- Visual Aid: Use pictures or diagrams of the Chokurei symbol as a reference. Place them in your healing space to focus your attention.
- Guided Visualization: Close your eyes and imagine the symbol glowing in front of you, radiating healing energy.

4. Drawing the Symbols

Chokurei:

- Physical Drawing: Use your hand to draw the symbol in the air or over the recipient's body. Start from the top of the vertical line and create the spiral.
- Paper Drawing: Before the session, draw the symbol on a piece of paper to focus your intention. You can place this drawing on or near the area needing healing.
- Body Drawing: Imagine drawing the symbol on the recipient's body, over the chakras, or the specific area that needs healing.

Practical Tips

- Combination: Use a combination of saying, thinking, seeing, and drawing for a more powerful effect. For example, say the symbol's name while visualizing and drawing it.
- Intention: Always set a clear intention before using the symbols. This focuses the energy and enhances the healing process.

- Practice: Regular practice with the symbols will strengthen your ability to use them effectively. Incorporate them into your daily routine to become more familiar and comfortable with their energy.

Practicing these techniques regularly will deepen your connection with the symbols and enhance your Reiki practice.

Used for Physical Healing

Chokurei *(Show Ku Ray)* Symbol

- *The forward 7 is used for general or whole-body healing*

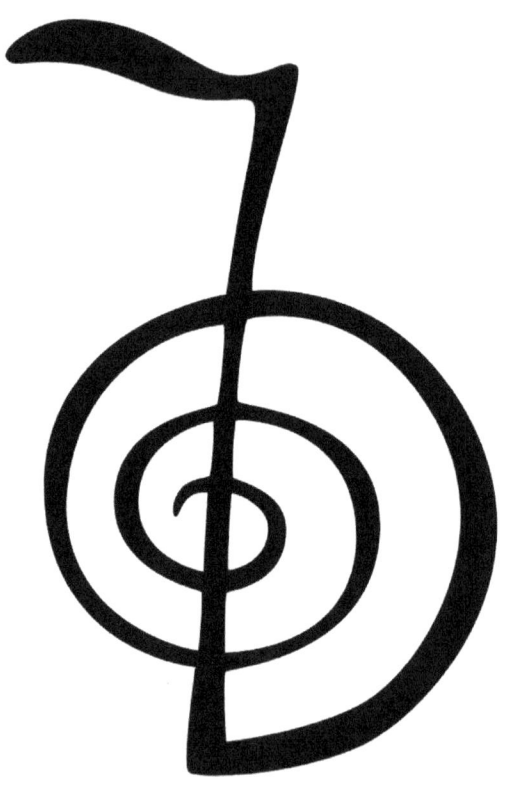

The Chokurei symbol, pronounced "Show Ku Ray," is one of the primary symbols used in Reiki, a form of energy healing. This symbol is often referred to as the Power Symbol and is used to enhance and focus energy during healing sessions.

Description

The Chokurei symbol resembles a stylized number seven with a spiral that wraps around the vertical line. The spiral starts from the top, making three and a half turns before ending at the base of the vertical line. There are different variations of the Chokurei, including a forward (clockwise) and a reverse (counterclockwise) version.

Uses in Physical Healing

Chokurei is primarily used for physical healing and serves several key functions:

1) Amplifying Energy: It acts like a light switch, turning on and amplifying the flow of Reiki energy. This helps to increase the effectiveness of the healing session.
2) Focus and Direction: By visualizing or drawing the symbol, practitioners can focus and direct energy to specific areas of the body that require healing.
3) Protection: It is also used to create a protective energy barrier around the healer and the recipient.

Application of the Forward 7

The forward version of Chokurei, which is drawn in a clockwise direction, is commonly used for general or whole-body healing. This version is believed to:

- Enhance the overall flow of energy throughout the body.
- Balance the body's energy systems, promoting overall physical health.
- Strengthen the immune system and aid in the body's natural healing processes.

How to Use Chokurei in a Healing Session

1) Preparation: Begin by centering yourself and connecting with the Reiki energy.
2) Drawing the Symbol: Use your hand or visualize the symbol in your mind. Draw the Chokurei over the area of the body you wish to heal. Start from the top of the vertical line, making three and a half spirals clockwise.
3) Intention: Focus on your intention to heal and direct energy to the area. Feel the energy amplifying and flowing into the recipient.
4) Channeling Energy: Continue to channel Reiki energy through your hands, allowing the symbol to guide and intensify the healing process.

The Chokurei symbol is a powerful tool in Reiki practice, enhancing the flow and focus of healing energy. Its forward (clockwise) version is particularly effective for general or whole-body healing, making it a versatile and essential component of Reiki sessions.

Chokurei (Show Ku Ray) Symbol: Backward 7

- *The backward 7 is used for specific or small areas.*

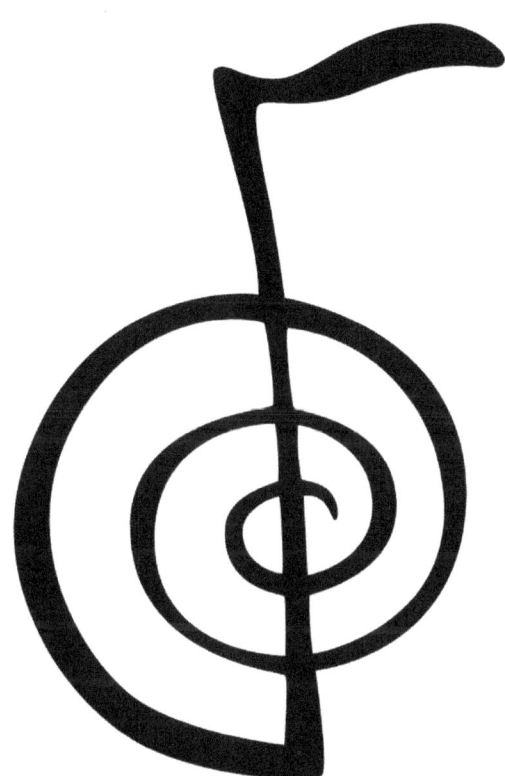

The Chokurei symbol, or "Show Ku Ray," has variations in its usage, one of which includes the backward or counterclockwise version. While the forward 7 is used for general or whole-body healing, the backward 7 is specifically applied for targeted or small-area healing.

Backward 7 Description

The backward version of Chokurei is drawn counterclockwise. Like the forward version, it consists of a vertical line with a spiral that wraps around it but in the opposite direction. This variation is used to concentrate the healing energy on specific, localized areas rather than dispersing it throughout the entire body.

Uses in Specific or Small Area Healing

The backward Chokurei symbol is particularly effective for:

1) Targeted Healing: It focuses Reiki energy on specific parts of the body that need concentrated healing, such as a wound, joint, or organ.
2) Precision: It allows the practitioner to direct the energy with precision, ensuring that the affected area receives the most benefit.
3) Intensifying Energy: By using the counterclockwise direction, the energy is believed to be intensified and condensed, making it more powerful for small areas.

How to Use the Backward 7 in a Healing Session

1) Preparation: Center yourself and connect with the Reiki energy, setting a clear intention for the healing session.
2) Drawing the Symbol: Visualize or draw the backward Chokurei over the specific area needing healing. Begin at the top of the vertical line and make the spiral counterclockwise.
3) Focusing Energy: Concentrate on channeling the Reiki energy into the small, targeted area. Visualize the energy becoming more concentrated and intense.

4) Healing Process: Hold your hands over the area, allowing the symbol to guide the energy flow precisely where needed.

Benefits of Using the Backward 7

1) Enhanced Healing for Localized Issues: This method is ideal for addressing localized pain, injuries, or illnesses, providing more effective healing to the affected area.
2) Energy Concentration: The backward spiral helps in concentrating the energy, making the healing process more powerful and effective for specific issues.
3) Complementary Use: It can be used in conjunction with the forward 7 symbol to provide both general and targeted healing in a single session.

The backward Chokurei symbol is an essential tool for Reiki practitioners, allowing for precise and focused healing. Its counterclockwise direction is particularly effective for small or specific areas, making it a versatile addition to the Reiki practice. By understanding and utilizing both the forward and backward versions of Chokurei, practitioners can offer comprehensive healing tailored to the needs of their clients.

Part "Two" Of Level 1 Attunement Meditation

Read this second part after drawing the symbols:

Meeting Your Reiki Master in Spirit

In a moment, I am going to ask you to experience yourself in a circular room in the center of your head, behind your eyes. This circular room has doors and windows that lead out from all sides. Each door, each window, leads to a different guide. One of the doors leads to your Reiki Master in Spirit. I'd like you now to imagine yourself in the circular room. Look around and experience all of the doors and windows. Ask yourself which door leads to your Reiki Master in Spirit. I want you to go over to it and stand before it. Ask to experience it in the most vivid form possible for you. You can see it....you can feel it... You can hear a description of it....or you can just know. What does the door look like?........How does it open?....Now, I want you to mark this door in some way so that you will always know that it leads to your Reiki Master in Spirit....You can put a symbol on it....you can write on it....anything at all....On the other side of this door is a corridor filled with golden light. I'd like you now to walk through this door....Stepping into the hallway....beginning to walk down it.... You may feel sunshine on you....you may see glittery, sparkling fairy dust....you may hear a tone or a melody....and you feel so wonderful that you're on you way to meet your Reiki Master in Spirit....Notice anything that's on the floors....the walls....or the ceiling.... Walk all the way down the hallway until you reach the next door....On the other side of this door is your Reiki Master in Spirit waiting to meet you.... We're going to make a conscious contract with your Reiki Master now....I want you to think of these three things after me... "My Reiki Master in Spirit has the highest level of integrity possible.". "My Reiki Master in Spirit comes in a form that I can easily accept.". "My Reiki Master in Spirit is at the highest level that I can readily communicate with.". And anything else that you would like to add that's specifically important to you....Now notice this door.... What is it made of?....How does it open?....Now walk through the door allowing your Reiki Master in Spirit to come in the most vivid form possible for you....so you can see it....hear it....feel it....or know that it is there....Greet it in a way that feels comfortable....you can give it a hug....say hello....bow....or shake its hand....Ask it what its name is....If it keeps changing form, ask it to choose one shape....Ask how it feels about you taking this step into Reiki....Please ask what its responsibilities are going to be in working with you....Thank it for assisting me in attuning you to 1st degree Reiki....Ask how you can get the most out of this Reiki attunement on body....mind....spirit....and emotional levels....Ask what you can do on each of those levels to enhance your experience....And anything else that you would like to ask....

I'd like you now to get ready to say goodbye....So go ahead....saying goodbye....embracing them....shaking their hand....bowing to them....whatever seems appropriate....Going back to the door and the corridor filled with golden light....shutting the door behind you....beginning to walk back down the hallway....feeling the sunlight on you....seeing the glittery fairy dust....hearing a tone or a melody....feeling so wonderful after having this experience....noticing anything on the floor....the walls....or the ceiling....Go all the way down to the end....back through the door, into the circular room....shutting the door behind you....

I'm going to in a moment have you take 3 deep breaths....as you breathe in, I would like you to envision that 1st degree Reiki energy going all the way down to a cellular level....as you breathe out, your intent is going to be to reprogram every cell down to the DNA to be attuned to 1st degree Reiki.....

So, breathing in that 1st degree of Reiki energy all the way down to the cellular level....Breathing out, programming every cell down to the DNA to be filled with 1st degree Reiki energy....Breathing in, 1st degree Reiki energy all the way down to the cellular level....Breathing out, every cell down to the DNA is attuned with 1st degree Reiki energy.One more time... Breathing in 1st degree Reiki energy all the way down to the cellular level....Breathing out, every cell is attuned to 1st degree Reiki energy.

Have each student talk about their experience *(who they met as their Reiki Master)*.

Reiki 21-Day Cleanse

There is no area of life that Reiki will not change and affect. It will assist in bringing goals and desires into manifested form. It will work at healing relationships. Wherever there is disparity and imbalance, the energy will reinstate order and stability.

Physical Purification: When Reiki is purifying the physical body, flu-like symptoms may be experienced. Minor discomforts include aching muscles, fever, headache, sore throat, excessive mucus, coughing, constipation, diarrhea, and other symptoms. As toxins are being released, odors in the urine and feces may change. Pressures or pains throughout the body, tingling, nausea, or spinning sensations may also be felt in the chakras as Reiki opens, cleanses, and balances them.

To lessen the effects, self-treatments should be done, long walks should be taken, the entire body should be exercised mildly, some deep breathing should be done, and lots of filtered water should be drank. Eat light, nourishing meals, which include fresh fruits and vegetables. Juicing or fasting is also beneficial.

Emotional Purification: As purification of the emotional body occurs, deeply held emotions may surface for no apparent reason: anger, frustration, grief, fear, sadness, and others. These emotions have been repressed or suppressed from earlier times in this lifetime or from past-life experiences. They are being released from the depths of your physical matrix — from the cellular level of body and mind.

Do not place blame on anyone for these feelings. Just experience them as they surface and let them go.

Place one hand on your forehead and the other on your navel to lessen the effects. Breathe in and visualize beautiful white light coming into your crown chakra, circling throughout your body, and collecting all the emotional remains. Then, breathe forcefully while visualizing the emotions released through your solar plexus chakra. Repeat until you feel calm. Take a long bath in sea salts, Epsom salts, or a combination of 1 pound each of sea salt and baking soda. This will relax you and help to cleanse your emotional body.

Mental Purification: When purification of the mental body occurs, old thought forms, behavior patterns and/or habits might surface. Addictive desires may resurface. Thoughts of judgment, blame, victimization, abuse, denial, self-destruction, self-pity, etc., may prevail. These issues are being healed on every level of your being, from this lifetime and others. Just take a look at them, let them go, and then change your thoughts willfully to those of a more positive nature.

To lessen the effects: Spend extra time doing self-Reiki treatments on the head positions. Do things that make you feel good: nurture and pamper yourself as you would a friend who was experiencing the same. Also, repeating positive affirmation mantras and listening to your favorite music eases the intensity of the potentially negative effects of the thoughts.

Spiritual Purification: When spiritual purification is in process, your beliefs may be shaken and challenged: beliefs in how the world operates, how relationships should be, about religion, what is important in life, etc. As this occurs, insights, revelations, and new understandings will become clear. These will be the building blocks of your newly forming and ever-changing spiritual foundation.

To lessen the effects: Talk to like-minded people about your experiences, read up-lifting books, listen to motivational tapes, and treat yourself with kindness. You are gaining new levels of understanding. During this process, you may feel lonely and perhaps fearful that you are going insane. Know that all is well and that this process is perfectly normal. Continue to do Reiki on yourself; this alone can and will move you through the purification process and bring you closer to that which you truly are: Divine Spirit, experiencing the physical realm of existence through the sensations of one magnificent vehicle — your body.

To lessen the effects, drink lots of filtered water, eat lots of raw fruit and vegetables, and exercise your whole body lightly (walking, swimming, etc.). Writing at the end of the day is an excellent way to clear your mind. Just write how you feel and why.

Reiki Self-Treatment Hand Positions

Reiki heals by flowing through the affected parts of the energy field and charging them with positive energy. It raises the vibratory level of the energy field in and around the physical body where the negative thoughts and feelings are attached. This causes the negative energy to break apart and fall away. In so doing, Reiki clears, straightens, and heals the energy pathways, thus allowing one's life force to flow healthily and naturally. The individual receiving the energy unconsciously draws the energy, and it naturally flows inside the body to the places where it is most needed. When there is a sufficiency, the energy transfer ends.

Because God-consciousness guides Reiki, it can never harm. It always knows what that person needs and will adjust itself to create the appropriate effect. One never needs to worry about whether to give Reiki or not. It is always helpful.

In addition, because the practitioner does not direct the healing and does not decide what to work on or what to heal, the practitioner is not in danger of taking on the client's karma. Because the practitioner is not doing the healing, it is also much easier for the ego to stay out of the way and allow God's presence to shine through.

The Reiki practitioner's energies are never depleted because it is a channeled healing. In fact, the Reiki consciousness considers both practitioner and client to be in need of healing, so both receive treatment. Because of this, giving treatment always increases one's energy and leaves one surrounded with loving feelings of well-being.

The Reiki practitioner is only the vehicle through which the energy is transmitted; the receiver is always responsible for allowing themselves to be healed.

RECEIVING INFORMATION WHILE GIVING A REIKI TREATMENT

Because you are at a higher intuitive space while channeling Reiki energy, you may receive flashes of intuitive knowledge about the patient and their condition or about changes that would improve their health. Just inform them of the information received, knowing they are responsible for their healing.

Types of Reiki Session Choice:

- Self Reiki Treatment

Reiki Self-Treatment

Self-healing is the crucial first step in becoming a Reiki Channel. You can only give others what you are willing to give yourself. Love and heal yourself first.

Daily self-treatments strengthen your health, and your life force's energy is recharged with each session.

You can do Reiki while you read, listen to music, or even watch television.

The more you use Reiki energy, the easier and stronger it will flow through you.

After receiving your first degree, your energy system must adjust to higher vibration levels. This energy will balance itself out in two to three months. Daily self-treatments are recommended to lessen the effects.

Reiki Breathing Exercise:

1. Make yourself comfortable by lying down or sitting, then close your eyes. Pay attention to the rhythm of your breathing.
2. Intuitively, place your hands on two of your chakra centers.
3. Now direct your breath (imagine it as the Universal Life Force Energy) consciously through your hands into the chakra centers. Notice the feeling of relaxation and peace as it gradually spreads throughout your body.
4. After about 5 min. Place your hands on two other chakra centers and again consciously breathe the Life Force Energy through your hands. Notice your
5. breathing. Did it change? Just allow yourself to let go of the "feeling of flowing."
6. Continue the hand placements until you cover all seven chakras. Be sure to focus on your breathing.
7. Slowly open your eyes. You will feel more relaxed, calm, and centered.

Quick Energizer:

1. Sit or lie down.
2. Place one hand on your Solar Plexus (3rd) Chakra.
3. Place your other hand directly under it, touching your stomach.
4. Close your eyes, relax your hands, and let your mind drift.
5. Stay in this position for 10-15 minutes.
6. Open your eyes. You will feel rejuvenated and refreshed with vital energy.

Sleep Help:

1. Lie on your back or side in a comfortable position.
2. Place one hand on your Spleen (2nd) Chakra and the other hand on your Third Eye (6th) Chakra. Notice your stomach rising and falling as you breathe.
3. Remain in that position until the Reiki energy generates a feeling of deep relaxation.

Reiki Self Treatment - Full Body

POSITIONS FOR SELF TREATMENT

1. Rub your hands together to bring the Reiki energy up to the surface of your hands.

2. Place one hand over your Solar Plexus (3rd) Chakra and one hand over your Spleen (2nd) Chakra.

3. Call upon your Reiki Master in Spirit and your Higher Self to assist you in this treatment. If you are attuned to 2nd or 3rd Degree, use the symbols at this time.

4. Ask that the Reiki energy flows through you at the highest level that benefits you right now.

5. Proceed with the hand positions described below:

THE HEAD

Position #1 Place your hands over your face.

Position #2 Place your hands on the top of your head, letting your middle fingers meet over the Crown (7th) Chakra.

Position #3 Cup your hands at the base of your head in either position.

Position #4 Form a "V" at your neck with the heals of your hands at the front.

THE FRONT

Position #1 Place your hands above your breast line, with your fingers touching in the middle.

Position #2 Place your hands over your breast with your fingertips meeting in the middle - Heart (4th) Chakra.

Position #3 Place both hands just above the navel - Solar Plexus (3rd) Chakra.

Position #4 Place both hands just below the navel - Spleen (2nd) Chakra.

Position #5 Place your hands toward the groin area in a "V" - Root (1st) Chakra.

THE BACK

Position #1 Place your hands around the back of your neck - Throat (5th) Chakra.

Position #2 Reach across your body and place your hands one at a time over the opposite shoulder.

Position #3 Reach your hands around your back, touching your fingers in the middle.

Position #4 Place your hands side to side just above your waist - Solar Plexus (3rd) Chakra.

Position #5 Place your hands downward over your tailbone - Root (1st) Chakra.

Position #6 Run the Reiki energy down your arms and out your fingers. Visualize the negative energy being grounded down into the earth.

Position #7 Run the Reiki energy down your legs and visualize the negative energy being grounded down into the earth.

Position #8 Place your hands at the bottom of your feet.

CLOSING A SELF TREATMENT

Say, "I ask that this Reiki energy continue to heal, harmonize, and balance my top with my bottom, my front with my back, my inside with my outside, my left with my right, and my yin with my yang. I also ask that this Reiki energy continue to heal, harmonize, and balance my body, mind, spirit, and emotions."

Reiki Level 1 – Apprentice Homework

1. What did you learn from each of the three degrees of Reiki?

   _____

   _____

   _____

2. What are the Four Miracles of Reiki?

   _____

   _____

   _____

   _____

3. What are the Five Principles of Reiki?

   _____

   _____

   _____

   _____

   _____

4. Describe your meditation meeting your Reiki Master in Spirit.

   _____

   _____

_____
_____
_____
_____
_____
_____
_____
_____
_____
_____
_____
_____
_____
_____
_____
_____
_____
_____
_____
_____
_____
_____
_____
_____
_____

5. Practice drawing the symbols and the self-reiki treatments.

REIKI LEVEL 2 – THE PRACTITIONER

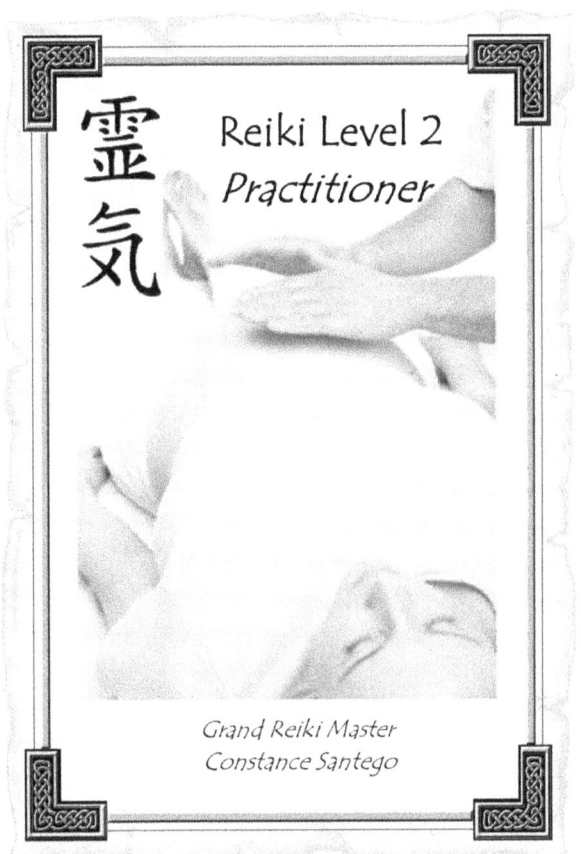

Reiki Level 2
Practitioner

Grand Reiki Master
Constance Santego

Level 2: Okuden

Okuden, meaning "Inner Teachings" or "Hidden Teachings,"
is the intermediate level of Reiki training. It introduces Reiki
symbols and advanced mental, emotional, and distant healing
techniques.

Reiki Level 2 Lesson Plan

Three – 3-hour live class

1st class

- Talk about mental and emotional healing

2nd part of 1st class
Listen and Subscribe

Part 1 https://youtu.be/qwPO1WVufUc

Part 2 https://youtu.be/59V4TLr69Jc

or *Read* the "Apprentice" Meditation

- o Read the 1st part of the meditation
- o Draw the level 2 symbols on each student
- o Finish the meditation
- Have each student talk about what they experienced

2nd and 3rd classes

- Practice giving and receiving
  - o On Each Other
  - o Distant Reiki Healing
  - o Mental Healing
  - o Emotional Healing
  - o Reiki on plants, children, and first aid
  - o Also, any of the other sessions taught in Secrets of a Healer – Magic of Reiki (Vol X)

Second Degree Reiki

Second Degree, Reiki attunement has a particular effect on the Chakra System. The attunement opens the Reiki channel between the Heart (4th) and the Crown (7th) Chakras. The lower Chakras, Root (1st) to the Solar Plexus (3rd), are adjusted to the higher Reiki energy during the 21-day cleansing period.

Second Degree, Reiki gives you a technique to help send healing energy in non-physical dimensions. This is referred to as Distant Healing".

Furthermore, you also learn a method for releasing deep emotional and mental problems. "Mental Healing" allows you to contact the subconscious and the higher self to bring about healing to the receiver via the spirit. Problems such as sleeplessness, addictions, depression, and nervousness are addressed by this method.

With Second Degree Reiki, your healing powers are greatly strengthened, which will stimulate the Third Eye (6th) Chakra. This will help develop your intuitive powers and enable you to receive messages much easier.

The confidential Reiki symbols and corresponding mantras increase your energy and generate a higher vibration within you. Using these symbols carries a great responsibility and should only be given if the Reiki Master knows you are responsible enough to work with them.

Your Reiki Master in Spirit

As in Reiki Level 1... Level 2 has an initiation of being attuned to the 2nd-degree energy as well.

Everyone is granted a Reiki Master in Spirit whose job is to help you facilitate a Reiki session. Your Reiki Master will be shown to you in your attunement to the Reiki energy. Most people keep their original Reiki Master, but I have had many students where the Master changes at different levels.

Meeting your Master is a very special experience; some feel wonderful tingles, some see beautiful colors and images, some hear music, and some just know it to be true. You will meet your Reiki Master through a meditation that will be read to you by your Reiki Master – In class or by YouTube – online. Your Reiki Master will always come to you in the form you can handle.

Enjoy the meditation.

LEVEL 2 MEDITATION FOR ATTUNEMENT

You have a choice:

1) Listen to the level 2 meditation on YouTube
   Part 1 https://youtu.be/qwPO1WVufUc
   Part 2 https://youtu.be/59V4TLr69Jc

Or

2) In class:
   a. Read the 1st part of the meditation,
   b. Draw the reiki symbols on each student's crown, heart chakras, and both palms. *(by holding Hui Yin and taking a Kidney Breath),*
   c. Read 2nd part of the meditation,
   d. Water Ritual (Draw the Symbols over the lemon water),
   e. Say the Raku Kei Affirmation

Part "One" Of Level 2 Attunement Meditation

Read this Meditation:

"Close your eyes....get comfortable.....get really relaxed..... Take a deep breath all the way down to the bottom of your lungs.....Now let your breath out slowly and completely.....Concentrate your attention behind your eyes....relax all the muscles in your

eyes..... Relax them completely..... Relax them so
much that they just won't open....And now that they
are relaxed, test them.....If they are relaxed they just
won't open.....Good.....Now take another deep
breath... Feel it as is expands every part of your
lungs.....Now exhale slowly and completely....Let that
same relaxation in your eye muscles go all the way
down to your toes.....Let go completely. Use your
imagination.....Now get ready to go beyond
yourself....From this point on, let all outside noises
increase your awareness of my voice....Let my voice be
your voice....Relax your toes
completely....Concentrate all your attention in your
feet. Let go....All the muscles in your
legs....concentrate on relaxing them now..... Your
lower legs... and your upper legs....Now concentrate
on relaxing your hips....your lower abdomen....and
your stomach....Relax your lower back....Relax your
chest....and your upper back....Not falling asleep.... Still
very much aware of everything that is going on....Able
to hear my voice clearly....Now relax all of the muscles
in your shoulders and neck....Relax your arms....all the
way down to your finger tips....Now concentrate on
relaxing your jaw... Relax it freely....Relax your
tongue....Now relax all of the muscles in your
face....your mouth....your eyes....your jaw....and your
forehead.... You're very deeply relaxed now....Not out
of touch with reality. Very much in tune with
everything I am saying. Completely aware of your
surroundings....just very, very deeply relaxed....Now,
you have reached a level of deep physical relaxation.

Let's concentrate on deep mental relaxation....For mental relaxation, I will count slowly from 100 to 98, so that you may double your relaxation with each number. When you reach 98, just let the number vanish. Here we go....100....Now double your relaxation, just let go....99....double again your relaxation, now even more relaxed....98....double one more time your relaxation....Now let the numbers vanish....Let them disappear.... This is a nice stage of relaxation. Not out of touch with reality....deeply in tune with everything I am saying....Completely aware of your surroundings....just very intent upon my voice....Allowing all noises to increase your attention....Repeat mentally the following affirmation:

In the province of the mind, I am unlimited.

(Repeat 6 more times)

The next time you go into meditation, you will go even deeper....It will work even better....faster....deeper.

Now, you will move to the higher side of yourself....Pure spirit....A being of light.... You are not your body. Concentrate your attention in your toes. Notice you have toes...and they are relaxed....but you are not your toes....Notice your feet now....and your lower legs....and your upper legs.... You are not these either....As you relax more and more, concentrate your attention on my voice....Notice you have hips, but you are not your hips....Notice your stomach....your chest....and your breathing....going in and out. You are not your stomach....and you are not your chest....and you are not your breathing. Notice your entire back....that's not who you are either. Notice your shoulders.... You're aware that they're there....they're yours....But you are not your shoulders....and you are not your arms either. Notice you have a neck....But you are not your neck.... Switch your consciousness to your jaw now....You are not your jaw. You are not your tongue....nor are you all the muscles in your face........including your nose....your eyes..........and your mouth.... You are not those....Notice your thoughts now....and you have thoughts....but you are not your thoughts....Go even deeper now....Give me your full attention.... Concentrate on my voice.

It is now time to raise your vibrational rate with feelings of love and strong positive thoughts. You may do this by surrounding yourself with a beautiful protective white light. This white light represents truth....forgiveness....your ideal concept of the Source, and all that is good. Picture this white light now starting to glow in your heart.

Allow this white light to glow within your heart....Let it increase. Feel its warmth and purity. Allow it to extend and to radiate out of your heart so that it envelops your body....Completely surrounding you in a cocoon of pure, vibrant white light.... This white light is the Source's perfect presence. You may actually see it....feel it....or sense it....but all you really have to do is to know it to be there. It will always be with you. You now have the protective white light around you so that your subconscious mind is only open to suggestions that are helpful and beneficial to you.....Bathe yourself in the white light....Notice that you are light.... You are pure spirit....A dearly beloved child of the Source....Beyond time and space. Feel your light extending....Emanate your light into infinity....

You are pure light....unconditional pure love....pure compassion....pure forgiveness. You are beyond the beyond....you are one with the universe.

Attune the Student:

1. *While the student holds their "Hui Yin," open their crown chakra with the Raku Symbol, then draw the Reiki Level 2 - Sei He Ki symbol into their crown, heart, and palms.*
2. *Now, the student takes a "Kidney Breath."*
3. *Close their crown with the Raku symbol...*
4. *Then, continue the second part of the meditation...*

Reiki Level 2 Symbols

Do not get to concerned about the variations of how the symbols are written. There are many Japanese symbols, and many Reiki Masters that use many other symbols.

A Japanese symbol is the same as a written word in ABC. It has the same power of intent. It will not matter if you draw the symbol, write the word, or say it aloud in English, Japanese, or any other language. It will all be the same to Your Reiki Master in Spirit. Pick your favorite way to have the intent of why you are going to use the ki energy.

Using Reiki Symbols:
Sei He Ki and Hon Sha Ze Sho Nen

Reiki symbols like Hon Sha Ze Sho Nen and Sei He Ki are powerful tools in energy healing, and there are multiple ways to use them during a session. Any of these methods can evoke the Reiki symbol and its energy. Here's how a person can say, think, see, or draw these symbols effectively:

Saying the Symbols

Sei He Ki (Say-Hey-Key):

- Verbal Invocation: Say "Sei He Ki" to focus on emotional and mental healing. Repeating the name helps in embedding the intention.
- Affirmation: Use phrases like "Sei He Ki, bring harmony and balance" or "Sei He Ki, help clear emotional blockages."

Hon Sha Ze Sho Nen (Hon-Sha-Zee-Show-Nen):

- Verbal Invocation: Say "Hon Sha Ze Sho Nen" out loud to activate its power for distant healing. Repeat it several times to enhance the energy.
- Affirmation: Use phrases like "Hon Sha Ze Sho Nen, connect me across time and space" or "Hon Sha Ze Sho Nen, send healing energy to [specific person/event]."

Thinking the Symbols

Sei He Ki:

- Mental Visualization: Visualize the Sei He Ki symbol clearly in your mind. Picture the vertical line and the intersecting wave-like line.
- Focus: Think about the symbol and its intent, imagining it balancing the emotional and mental energies.

Hon Sha Ze Sho Nen:

- Mental Visualization: Picture the Hon Sha Ze Sho Nen symbol in your mind's eye. Imagine drawing it mentally, starting from the top and following the specific kanji pattern.
- Focus: Concentrate on the symbol and its purpose, visualizing it and connecting you to the recipient across time and space.

Seeing the Symbols

Sei He Ki:

- Visual Aid: During sessions, keep images of the Sei He Ki symbol nearby. Look at these images to help visualize the symbol in your mind.
- Guided Visualization: With your eyes closed, see the symbol in your mind, glowing and bringing harmony to the emotional and mental state.

Hon Sha Ze Sho Nen:

- Visual Aid: Use pictures or diagrams of the Hon Sha Ze Sho Nen symbol as a reference. Place them in your healing space to focus your attention.
- Guided Visualization: Close your eyes and imagine the symbol glowing in front of you, radiating healing energy across the distance.

Drawing the Symbols

Sei He Ki:

- Physical Drawing: Draw the symbol in the air or over the recipient's body with your hand. Start with the vertical line and then add the wave-like intersecting line.
- Paper Drawing: Sketch the symbol on paper to set your intention. Use this drawing as a visual aid during the healing session.
- Body Drawing: Visualize drawing the symbol on the recipient's forehead, heart, or any area associated with emotional or mental issues.

Hon Sha Ze Sho Nen:

- Physical Drawing: Use your hand to draw the symbol in the air or over the recipient's body. Start from the top of the kanji pattern and draw each part with intention.
- Paper Drawing: Before the session, draw the symbol on a piece of paper to focus your intention. Place this drawing on or near the area needing distant healing.
- Body Drawing: Imagine drawing the symbol on the recipient's body, over the chakras, or the specific area that needs healing, even if they are far away.

Benefits of Using Reiki Symbols

- Enhanced Healing Power: Using Reiki symbols can amplify the healing energy, making the session more effective for the recipient.
- Versatility: Reiki symbols allow for healing across distances (Hon Sha Ze Sho Nen) and target specific emotional and mental issues (Sei He Ki), providing a wide range of applications.
- Deepened Intention: The use of symbols helps practitioners focus their intentions more clearly, enhancing the healing session's overall effectiveness.
- Emotional and Mental Balance: Sei He Ki specifically aids in balancing emotions and clearing mental blockages, promoting mental clarity and emotional stability.
- Connection Across Time and Space: Hon Sha Ze Sho Nen allows for distant healing, making it possible to send Reiki energy to individuals, events, or situations regardless of their physical location.

- Holistic Healing: Combining the use of these symbols can address physical, emotional, mental, and spiritual aspects of well-being, providing a more comprehensive healing experience.

Practical Tips

Combination: Use a combination of saying, thinking, seeing, and drawing for a more powerful effect. For example, say the symbol's name while visualizing and drawing it.

Intention: Always set a clear intention before using the symbols. This focuses the energy and enhances the healing process.

Practice: Regular practice with the symbols will strengthen your ability to use them effectively. Incorporate them into your daily routine to become more familiar and comfortable with their energy.

Practicing these techniques regularly will deepen your connection with the symbols and enhance your Reiki practice.

Sei He Ki *(Say Hey Key)* Reiki Symbol

Sei He Ki, pronounced "Say Hey Key," is another significant Reiki symbol primarily used for emotional and mental healing. It is often referred to as the Harmony Symbol or the Mental/Emotional Symbol. This symbol helps to balance the right and left sides of the brain, promoting mental clarity and emotional stability.

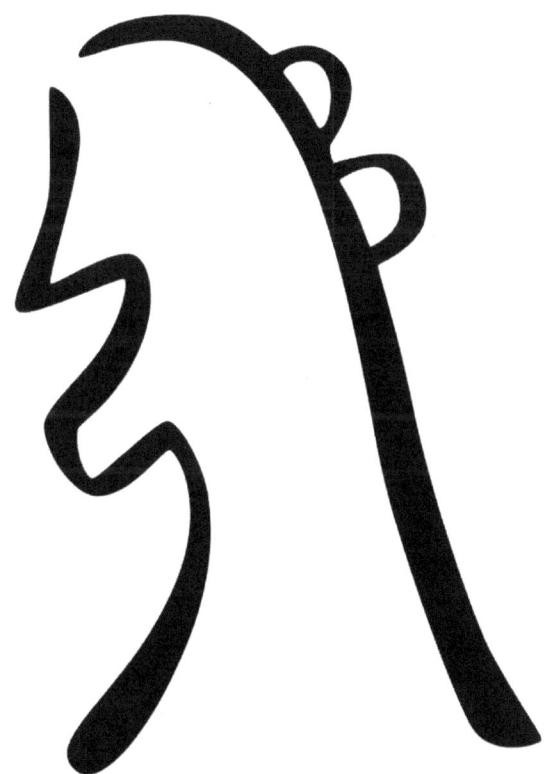

Description

The Sei He Ki symbol looks like a wave or a sideways lightning bolt that is intersected by a vertical line. Some interpret it as representing the brain's two hemispheres or the harmony between mind and body. The symbol is intricate and can be visualized or drawn during a Reiki session to invoke its healing properties.

Uses in Emotional and Mental Healing

Sei He Ki is specifically used for:

1) Emotional Balance: It helps to release emotional distress, promoting peace and calm. It can be used to address issues such as anxiety, depression, and emotional trauma.
2) Mental Clarity: It aids in clearing mental blockages enhancing focus and concentration. This is particularly useful for those struggling with stress, confusion, or mental fatigue.
3) Addictions and Negative Habits: It supports breaking free from negative habits and addictions by addressing the underlying emotional and mental causes.
4) Relationships: It can be used to heal and improve relationships by fostering better communication and understanding.

How to Use Sei He Ki in a Healing Session

1) Preparation: As with any Reiki session, begin by centering yourself and connecting with the Reiki energy. Set a clear intention for emotional or mental healing.
2) Drawing the Symbol: Visualize or draw the Sei He Ki symbol either on the client's body, in the air, or mentally. Start with the vertical line, then draw the wave-like horizontal line intersecting it.

3) Focusing on the Issue: Concentrate on the specific emotional or mental issue that needs healing. Hold the intention clearly in your mind.
4) Channeling Energy: Channel the Reiki energy through your hands, allowing the Sei He Ki symbol to guide the energy to the areas of the brain or body where it is needed.
5) Affirmations and Visualization: Use positive affirmations and visualization techniques to enhance the healing process. Imagine the negative emotions or thoughts being cleared away and replaced with positive, harmonious energy.

Benefits of Using Sei He Ki

- Emotional Release: Helps in releasing pent-up emotions, providing a sense of relief and calm.
- Mental Clarity: Improves focus and mental sharpness, aiding in better decision-making and problem-solving.
- Stress Reduction: Alleviates stress and anxiety, promoting overall mental well-being.
- Enhanced Relationships: Fosters better interpersonal relationships by clearing emotional blockages and improving communication.

Practical Applications

- Daily Practice: Practitioners can use Sei He Ki on themselves daily to maintain emotional and mental balance.
- Healing Sessions: Incorporate Sei He Ki into Reiki sessions to help clients deal with emotional and mental issues.

- Distance Healing: The symbol can be used in distance healing to send emotional and mental healing energy to someone not physically present.
- Affirmations: Combine the symbol with positive affirmations for enhanced effects.

Sei He Ki is a powerful symbol in Reiki, which is dedicated to emotional and mental healing. By using this symbol, practitioners can help clients achieve emotional balance, mental clarity, and overall well-being. Understanding and effectively utilizing Sei He Ki can significantly enhance the healing process, providing profound benefits for both the practitioner and the recipient.

The Sei He Ki Reiki Mantra

Sei He Ki (pronounced "Say-Hay-Key") is one of the sacred symbols used in Reiki Level 2 (Okuden). It is known as the emotional and mental healing symbol, helping to balance the mind and emotions. The mantra associated with Sei He Ki enhances its healing power and effectiveness.

Meaning and Purpose of Sei He Ki

- Emotional Balance: Sei He Ki is primarily used to heal emotional and mental issues. It helps release emotional blockages, reduce stress, and promote mental clarity.
- Harmony and Protection: This symbol brings harmony to emotional and mental states and provides protection against negative energies and influences.
- Enhancement of Memory: Sei He Ki can also be used to enhance memory and improve the learning process.

How to Use the Sei He Ki Mantra

1. Drawing the Symbol:
    *   The Sei He Ki symbol is drawn in a specific way, usually starting with a vertical line, followed by a series of wave-like lines intersecting it. Visualizing or physically drawing the symbol while using the mantra can enhance its power.
2. Chanting the Mantra:
    *   Repetition: Repeat the mantra "Sei He Ki" either silently or out loud. Chanting it multiple times helps to activate the symbol's energy and focus your intention.
    *   Focus: As you chant, focus on the area needing emotional or mental healing. Visualize the healing energy flowing into this area, bringing balance and harmony.
3. Meditation:
    *   Prepare for Meditation: Sit or lie down in a comfortable position. Close your eyes and take a few deep breaths to relax.
    *   Visualize the Symbol: Visualize the Sei He Ki symbol in your mind's eye. Imagine it glowing with bright light.
    *   Chant the Mantra: Begin chanting "Sei He Ki" slowly and deliberately. Allow the sound to resonate within you, feeling the energy it brings.
    *   Intentional Focus: Direct the energy of the mantra towards your emotional and mental state or toward a specific situation or person needing healing.
4. Healing Sessions:

- Self-Healing: Place your hands on the areas of your body where you feel emotional or mental discomfort. Chant "Sei He Ki" and visualize the symbol entering and healing these areas.
- Healing Others: When providing Reiki to others, draw the Sei He Ki symbol over the recipient's body or the affected area. Chant the mantra while visualizing the symbol's energy flowing into the person, bringing emotional and mental balance.

Benefits of Using the Sei He Ki Mantra

1. Emotional Release:
   - Helps release stored emotional pain and trauma, promoting emotional freedom and well-being.
2. Mental Clarity:
   - Reduces mental clutter and enhances clarity of thought, aiding in decision-making and problem-solving.
3. Stress Reduction:
   - Calms the mind and reduces stress, fostering a sense of peace and relaxation.
4. Enhanced Healing:
   - Amplifies the healing effects of Reiki, especially in addressing emotional and mental issues.
5. Spiritual Protection:
   - Provides a shield against negative energies, protecting your emotional and mental states.

By incorporating the Sei He Ki mantra into your Reiki practice, you can significantly enhance your ability to address emotional and mental imbalances, providing a deeper and more holistic healing experience.

The primary mantra associated with the Sei He Ki symbol in Reiki is simply "Sei He Ki," which is chanted to activate the symbol's energy and intention. However, practitioners often use affirmations and additional phrases to deepen their connection with the symbol and enhance its healing effects. Here are some examples of how you can expand on the Sei He Ki mantra with associated affirmations:

Expanded Sei He Ki Mantras and Affirmations

1. Basic Mantra:
    a. "Sei He Ki": Chanting the name of the symbol itself. This is the most direct and commonly used mantra.
2. Affirmations for Emotional Healing:
    a. "Sei He Ki, bring harmony and balance to my emotions."
    b. "Sei He Ki, help release my emotional pain and trauma."
    c. "Sei He Ki, fill me with peace and emotional stability."
3. Affirmations for Mental Clarity:
    a. "Sei He Ki, clear my mind and enhance my focus."
    b. "Sei He Ki, bring clarity and insight into my thoughts."
    c. "Sei He Ki, help me to think clearly and make wise decisions."
4. Affirmations for Protection:
    a. "Sei He Ki, protect me from negative energies and influences."

b. "Sei He Ki, shield my mind and emotions from harm."
c. "Sei He Ki, create a barrier of light around me."
5. Affirmations for Harmony and Balance:
   a. "Sei He Ki, balance my emotional and mental energies."
   b. "Sei He Ki, harmonize my thoughts and feelings."
   c. "Sei He Ki, bring equilibrium to my inner world."

How to Use These Mantras and Affirmations

1. Meditation:
   a. Prepare: Find a quiet space, sit comfortably, and close your eyes.
   b. Visualize: Picture the Sei He Ki symbol in your mind's eye, glowing with light.
   c. Chant and Affirm: Begin with chanting "Sei He Ki," and then incorporate any of the above affirmations that resonate with your needs. For example, chant "Sei He Ki" three times, followed by "Sei He Ki, bring harmony and balance to my emotions."
2. During Reiki Sessions:
   a. Self-Healing: Place your hands on the parts of your body where you feel emotional or mental distress—Chant "Sei He Ki" followed by a relevant affirmation.
   b. Healing Others: While giving Reiki to others, draw the Sei He Ki symbol over their body or the affected area. Chant "Sei He Ki" and silently

or aloud state an affirmation that addresses
their needs.

3. Daily Practice:
    a. Morning Routine: Start your day by chanting
        "Sei He Ki" and reciting an affirmation to set a
        positive and balanced tone for the day.
4. Night Routine: End your day with a Sei He Ki
    meditation, focusing on releasing any emotional or
    mental stress accumulated throughout the day.

Example Mantra Practice

1. Begin with Centering:
    a. Sit comfortably, close your eyes, and take
        several deep breaths to center yourself.
2. Invoke the Symbol:
    a. Visualize the Sei He Ki symbol glowing in front
        of you or within you.
3. Chant the Mantra:
    a. Chant "Sei He Ki" slowly and deliberately,
        allowing the sound to resonate within you.
4. Add Affirmations:
    a. Follow the chant with an affirmation. For
        example:
    b. "Sei He Ki" (repeat three times)
    c. "Sei He Ki, bring harmony and balance to my
        emotions."
5. Integrate the Energy:
    a. Sit in silence for a moment, allowing the
        energy and affirmation to integrate into your
        being.

Incorporating these extended mantras and affirmations can deepen your practice with the Sei He Ki symbol, enhancing its benefits for emotional healing, mental clarity, and protection. This approach makes your Reiki sessions more powerful and tailored to your specific needs or those of your clients.

Hon Sha Ze Sho Nen:
The Distant Healing Symbol in Reiki

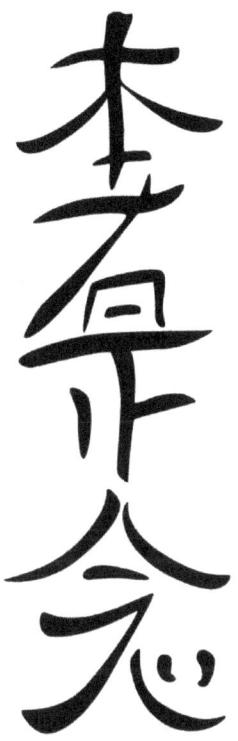

Hon Sha Ze Sho Nen, which is specifically associated with distant healing.

What is Hon Sha Ze Sho Nen?

Hon Sha Ze Sho Nen (pronounced as "Hon-Sha-Zee-Show-Nen") is one of the key symbols in Reiki, introduced in the second degree (Level 2) of Reiki training. This symbol is used to send healing energy across time and space, making it possible to perform Reiki healing on someone who is not physically present.

Meaning and Translation

The exact translation of Hon Sha Ze Sho Nen varies, but it is often interpreted as "The Divine in me honors the Divine in you" or "No past, no present, no future." It signifies the transcendence of time and space, allowing the practitioner to send healing energy to anyone, anywhere, at any time.

Appearance of the Symbol

Hon Sha Ze Sho Nen is typically depicted as a series of Japanese kanji characters combined in a unique pattern. The symbol is complex and requires practice to be drawn correctly. Each part of the symbol has specific meanings and represents different aspects of distant healing.

Uses of Hon Sha Ze Sho Nen

1. Distant Healing: The primary use of Hon Sha Ze Sho Nen is to send Reiki energy to someone who is not physically present. This can include people in different locations, situations in the past or future, or even to oneself.
2. Healing Past Trauma: By sending Reiki energy to past events, practitioners believe they can help heal emotional wounds and traumas, which can positively affect the present.
3. Future Events: Reiki energy can also be sent to future events, such as an upcoming surgery, job interview, or any situation where positive energy and outcomes are desired.

Situations and Relationships: Hon Sha Ze Sho Nen can be used to send healing energy to situations or relationships that need balance and harmony, helping to resolve conflicts and improve understanding.

How to Use Hon Sha Ze Sho Nen

1. Activate the Symbol: Begin by drawing or visualizing the symbol in your mind. Reiki practitioners are often taught to draw the symbol in the air or on their hands before starting a session.
2. Set Your Intention: Clearly state your intention for the healing session. This could be a specific person, event, or situation to which you wish to send energy.
3. Use Visualization: Visualize the person, event, or situation you are sending healing energy to. Imagine the Reiki energy flowing from your hands and reaching the intended recipient, enveloping them in healing light.
4. Invoke the Symbol: Say the symbol's name, "Hon Sha Ze Sho Nen," either out loud or silently, to invoke its power and connect with the distant recipient.
5. Perform the Healing: Continue to send Reiki energy for as long as you feel it is necessary. Trust your intuition to guide the flow of energy.

Benefits of Using Hon Sha Ze Sho Nen

- Flexibility: Allows healing sessions to be conducted without the need for physical presence, making it accessible to people who are far away or unable to attend in person.
- Time Transcendence: Enables healing of past traumas and future anxieties, promoting overall emotional and mental well-being.

- Empowerment: Empowers practitioners to provide support and healing to a broader range of people and situations, expanding the reach of Reiki's benefits.
- Hon Sha Ze Sho Nen is a powerful symbol in Reiki, offering the ability to send healing energy across time and space. Its use can significantly enhance a practitioner's ability to provide comprehensive healing, addressing physical ailments and emotional and mental challenges. By understanding and using this symbol, Reiki practitioners can extend their healing practice globally, helping others regardless of distance.

Part "Two" Of Level 2 Attunement Meditation

Read this second part after drawing the symbols:

Meeting Your Reiki Master in Spirit

In a moment, I am going to ask you to experience yourself in a circular room in the center of your head, behind your eyes. This circular room has doors and windows that lead out from all sides. Each door, each window, leads to a different guide. One of the doors leads to your Reiki Master in Spirit. I'd like you now to imagine yourself in the circular room. Look around and experience all of the doors and windows. Ask yourself which door leads to your Reiki Master in Spirit. I want you to go over to it and stand before it. Ask to experience it in the most vivid form possible for you. You can see it....you can feel it... you can hear a description of it....or you can just know. What does the door look like?........How does it open?....Now, I want you to mark this door in some way so that you will always know that it leads to your Reiki Master in Spirit....You can put a symbol on it....you can write on it....anything at all....On the other side of this door is a corridor filled with golden light. I'd like you now to walk through this door....Stepping into the hallway....beginning to walk down it.... You may feel sunshine on you....you may see glittery, sparkling fairy dust....you may hear a tone or a melody....and you feel so wonderful that you're on your way to meet your Reiki Master in Spirit....Notice anything that's on the floors....the walls....or the ceiling.... Walk all the way down the hallway until you reach the next door....On the other side of this door is your Reiki Master in Spirit waiting to meet you.... We're going to make a conscious contract with your Reiki Master now....I want you to think of these three things after me... "My Reiki Master in Spirit has the highest level of integrity possible.". "My Reiki Master in Spirit comes in a form that I can easily accept.". "My Reiki Master in Spirit is at the highest level that I can readily communicate with.". And anything else that you would like to add that's specifically important to you....Now notice this door.... What is it made of?....How does it open?....Now walk through the door allowing your Reiki Master in Spirit to come in the most vivid form possible for you....so you can see it....hear it....feel it....or know that it is there....Greet it in a way that feels comfortable....you can give it a hug....say hello....bow....or shake its hand....Ask it what its name is....If it keeps changing form, ask it to choose one shape....Ask how it feels about you taking this step into Reiki....Please ask what its responsibilities are going to be in working with you....Thank it for assisting me in attuning you to 1st degree Reiki....Ask how you can get the most out of this Reiki attunement on body....mind....spirit....and emotional levels....Ask what you can do on each of those levels to enhance your experience....And anything else that you would like to ask....

I'd like you now to get ready to say goodbye....So go ahead....saying goodbye....embracing them....shaking their hand....bowing to them....whatever seems appropriate....Going back to the door and the corridor filled with golden light....shutting the door behind you....beginning to walk back down the hallway....feeling the sunlight on you....seeing the glittery fairy dust....hearing a tone or a melody....feeling so wonderful after having this experience....noticing anything on the floor....the walls....or the ceiling....Go all the way down to the end....back through the door, into the circular room....shutting the door behind you....

I'm going to in a moment have you take three deep breaths....as you breathe in, I would like you to envision that 2nd degree Reiki energy going all the way down to a cellular level....as you breathe out, your intent is going to be to reprogram every cell down to the DNA to be attuned to 2nd degree Reiki.....

So, breathing in that 2nd degree of Reiki energy all the way down to the cellular level....Breathing out, programming every cell down to the DNA to be filled with 2nd degree Reiki energy....Breathing in, 2nd degree Reiki energy all the way down to the cellular level....Breathing out, every cell down to the DNA attuned with 2nd degree Reiki energy...One more time... Breathing in 2nd degree Reiki energy all the way down to the cellular level....Breathing out, every cell is attuned to 2nd degree of Reiki energy.

Have each student talk about their experience *(who they met as their Reiki Master)*.

A Reiki Treatment On A Client

Types of Reiki Session Choices:

1. Physical Healing
2. Distant Healing
   a) Visualization
   b) Full Body Absentee Treatment Hand
   c) Sandwich Treatment
3. Mental Healing
4. Emotional Healing

How A Treatment Is Given:

While the client is lying fully clothed, the practitioner first fills their own body with universal life force energy, then "sends" (actually, the client draws from the practitioner the amount of Reiki energy that is needed at that time) the energy out through their hands into the client's body.

Although the practitioner performs a basic pattern of hand placements on the front and back of the client's body, Reiki has its own "intelligence" and seeks out the cause and site of dysfunction, healing and relieving it.

Aromatherapy, candles, and soothing music are often used to enhance the Reiki treatment. Crystals and stones are also known to have powerful healing properties and can be used during a Reiki treatment.

A full body treatment takes approximately 1 hour.

Before You Give A Treatment:

Be sure that your client is comfortable; provide pillows, one for their head and one under their knees, and have a blanket available in case they are cold.

You may need to demonstrate the hand positions you will be using during the treatment to the client. Tell them about the possible 21-day cleanse that they will experience. Not everyone has the same symptoms. In my experience, only a few people ever experience adverse side effects. I tell the client it is possible but not likely.

Explain to them that during the treatment, they may experience -nothing at all- relaxation, warmth, coolness, tingling, energy running through their body, emotional release, and insight into past life experiences. *Ensure they know you have no control over what they experience. They receive what is needed at that time.*

If touching the client, be aware of how much hand pressure you use. Your hands should be relaxed and gently placed on the client's body. You do not have to touch the client to have the Reiki energy work.

Tell them that you are just the healing channel and that they are responsible for their healing.

Reiki Procedure

1. Have your client lie face up on the massage table. Place a pillow behind their knees if they would like. Cover them with a blanket. Some people like a small eye pillow. If you are going to use one place, a folded Kleenex should be over their eyes first for sanitary purposes.
2. Center yourself:
    a. Do some deep breathing or whatever method you use to center and calm yourself.
    b. Rub your hands together - this brings the Reiki energy up to the surface of your hands.
    c. Call upon their higher self or healing guide, your higher self, and your Reiki Master in Spirit to assist you in this healing.

When you have been attuned to 2nd Degree or 3rd Degree Reiki, you will also be using the appropriate symbol. Just think about it, say it out loud, draw it, or whatever you feel comfortable with.

-If you are doing Physical healing, use the Chokurei

-If you are using Distant healing, use the Hon Sha Ze Sho Nen

-If you are doing Mental or Emotional healing, use the Sei He Ki

-if you are doing Spiritual healing, use the Dai Ko Myo

   d. To yourself, say, "I ask that this Reiki energy flows through me at the highest level that is beneficial for my client and me."

HAND POSITIONS FOR TREATING A CLIENT

> e. Follow the hand positions for front and back, allowing the energy to flow for approx. Three minutes at each position.

Leave one hand on or hovering over the client at all times. If you disconnect, rub your hands together again, place them on the chakra you were doing, and use the appropriate symbols if you are at 2nd or 3rd Degree.

THE FRONT OF THE BODY

Position #1 Hands cupped gently over the eyes - Third Eye (6th) Chakra.

Position #2 Hands on top of the head - Crown (7th) Chakra.

Position #3 Hands under the head.

Position #4 Hands cupped gently hovering the throat - Throat Chakra (5th)

Position #5 Hands placed in a "V" flat on or hovering over the upper chest.

Position #6 Hands placed over each shoulder, cupping them.

Position #7 Arms (each individually) Imagine running the Reiki energy from their shoulder to their wrist.

Position #8 Sandwich their hand between yours - sweep the negative energy out of their fingers: repeat #7 & #8 on the other arm.

Position #9 Hover your hands over their heart – Heart (4th) Chakra.

Position #10 Hover hands, one in front of the other just above the navel *(belly button)* – Solar Plexus (3rd) Chakra.

Position #11 Hover hands, one in front of the other, just below the navel – Spleen (2nd) Chakra.

Position #12 Hover your hands in a "V" starting at the waist.

Position #13 Hover your hands above the genitals – Root (1st) Chakra.

Position #14 Imagine running Reiki energy from their hip down one leg to their ankle.

Position #15 Sandwich the feet between your hands and sweep the negative energy away. Repeat #14 & #15 on the other leg.

THE BACK OF THE BODY

RECONNECT AT THE SOLAR PLEXUS (2nd) AND SPLEEN(3rd) CHAKRAS, USE THE SYMBOLS AT THIS TIME.

Position #1 "Mental Clearing" Hover one hand on top of the Crown (7th) Chakra.

> Place the other hand across the occipital ridge, perpendicular to the first hand.

> Then, draw the RAKU, CHOKUREI & SEHEKI symbols over the Crown Chakra, gently touching the Crown Chakra after each symbol.

> Say the "SEI HE KI" mantra three times.

Then, say to your client, "Take a couple of deep breaths, and when you breathe out, let go of any limitations, past or present".

Position #2 Hover your hands over the back of the neck, your fingers touching, forming a pyramid.

Position #3 Hover your hands downward from shoulders in a "V," touching the index fingers.

Position #4 Hover your hands, one in front of the other, over the Heart (4th) Chakra.

Position #5 Hover your hands, one in front of the other, over the Solar Plexus (3rd) Chakra.

Position #6 Hover your hands, one in front of the other, over the Spleen (2nd) Chakra.

Position #7 Hover your hands, in a "V" over the buttocks.

Position #8 Imagine running Reiki energy from their hip down one leg to their ankle.

Position #9 Hover your hands at the bottom of their feet.

ENDING A REIKI TREATMENT ON A CLIENT

Before you take your hands off a client, it is suggested that you say and do the following:

1. "I ask that this Reiki energy continue to heal, harmonize, and balance your top with your bottom, your front with your back, your inside with your outside, your left with your right, and your yin with your yang."

2. "I also ask that this Reiki energy continue to heal, harmonize, and balance your body, mind, spirit, and emotions if that is for your highest good."

To disconnect your energy from theirs, imagine a bubble out in front of you.

Ask that any energy that you inadvertently took on go into that bubble.

Dissolve the bubble into neutralized energy (visualize static on a TV screen) and send it down to the earth's center. *This is a way of making it clear to the universe that you, as the practitioner, are not intentionally or unintentionally taking on your clients "stuff."*

3. Silently thank your client's Higher Self, your Higher Self, and your Reiki Master in Spirit.
4. Remove your hands from your client.
5. Explain to your client that the Reiki energy is still inside them and that they should continue to allow it to heal down to the cellular level. *If you received any intuitive knowledge during the session, you can tell them about it.*
6. Remind them about the possible 21-day cleanse and advise them to drink plenty of fresh water to help release toxins.
7. Explain that it's normal to feel a little light-headed after the treatment. *Have some water on hand for them to drink, and give them a few minutes to get centered.*

8. Also, tell them to feel free to call if anything surfaces from the session that they would like to talk about.

Distant Healing

You can imagine the person lying on your massage table in full size, or have your hands approximately a foot apart and image the person is between your palms, or image the person tiny between your prayer-held hands, or have a teddy bear or doll be a surrogate of the person or even a photograph of the person can be used.

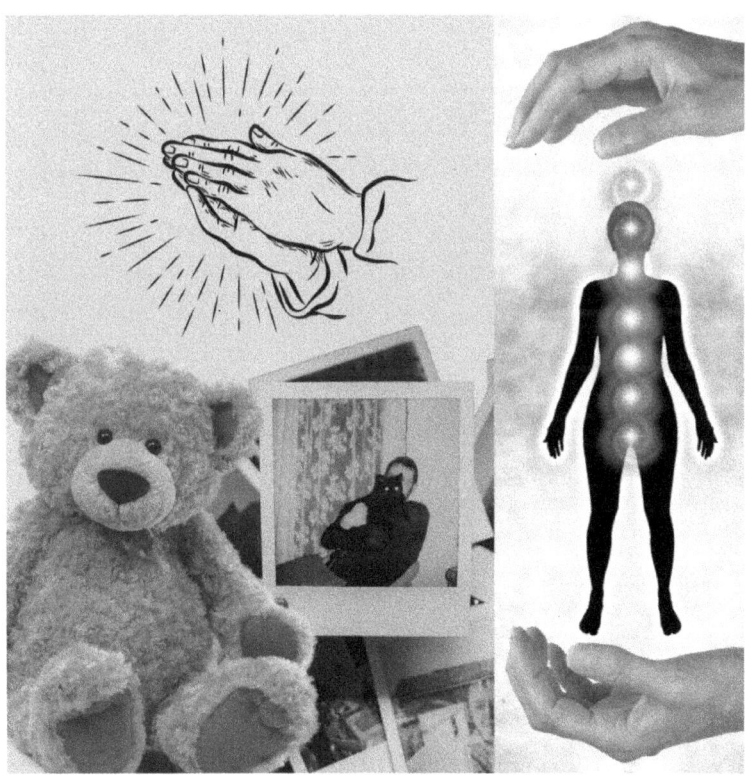

Remember that you are not trying to create a specific result. Know that Reiki will work for the highest good of all concerned.

Never assume that another being wants to be healed. If the recipient does not accept the Reiki energy, it will be returned to you.

Always honor the energy and your intention.

Distant Healing Visualization:

1. Fill your heart with unconditional love and acceptance. Put your hands over your heart until you feel totally peaceful and connected with this energy.

2. Imagine that you are full of a golden light that charges your whole body and radiates from it. This light encases your body like a protective shell.

3. Now, "sense" the person to whom you want to send some healing. If you are attuned to the Second Degree, you can use the symbols for distant healing at this point. Once the person appears in your mind's eye, "he, she, or they" are surrounded by golden light.

4. Now, through visualization/imagination, you send the light energy from the palms of your hands to the person to whom you are being treated. Imagine two laser-like beams of light flowing as healing energy from your palms into the receiver's body. You can also imagine sending loving and healing thoughts to that person.

5. To break the connection between you and the receiver, imagine the light that encompasses both of you to be slowly dispersed into nothingness.

Full Body Absentee Treatment

1. Call upon the client's spirit to be present.

2. Imagine them about two feet tall.

3. Call upon their Healing Guide and Higher Self and your Higher Self and Reiki Master in Spirit to assist you in facilitating this treatment.

4. Trace HON SHA ZA SHO NEN over their torso. Do a RAKU and CHOKUREI over their navel.

5. Ask that the Reiki energy flows through you at the highest possible level that benefits you and your client.

6. Proceed with the usual hand positions. Note: since they are smaller, it will take fewer hand positions to cover the entire body.

7. Send their spirit back to their body.

8. Thank the client's Healing Guide and Higher Self and your Higher Self and Reiki Master in Spirit.

9. To disconnect, imagine a bubble out in front of you. Ask that any of your client's energy you inadvertently took go into that bubble. Dissolve the bubble into neutralized energy and send it down to the earth's center.

The Hand Sandwich Treatment

It is used when you do not have time for a whole body treatment."

1. Ask your clients for permission.

2. Imagine them palm-size, and visualize them lying down in the palm of your hand.

3. Call upon their Higher Self and Healing Guide and your Higher Self and Reiki Master in Spirit to assist you in facilitating this treatment.

4. Then say, "I ask that this Reiki energy flows through me at the highest level that benefits me and ____(client)."

5. Do HON SHA ZA SHO NEN, RAKU, CHOKUREI, and SEHEKI symbols above the visualized client.

6. Place your hand over the hand that you visualize them in. Keep this position for 10 to 15 minutes.

7. In closing, the treatment is followed by the closing for the full body treatment.

Using the technique of "Distant Healing," you can send healing and light into specific problem areas:

In case of general unrest or during disasters or wars, you can send Reiki to the entire World or concentrate on a specific area. "Reiki together in a group is a good idea because it creates a more powerful energy field."

Difficult or unresolved situations can be resolved for yourself or others.

You can also work on and heal past traumatic events from your life, such as childhood wounds, abuse, etc.

"Distant Healing" also works well on animals.

Reiki Practitioner's Mind and Personal Issues During Mental or Emotional Reiki Sessions

Practitioners of Reiki play a crucial role in channeling healing energy to their clients. However, their mental and emotional state can significantly impact the session's effectiveness. Here's how practitioners can manage their mind and personal issues while performing mental or emotional Reiki sessions.

Importance of Practitioner's Mental and Emotional State

1. Energy Transfer
   - Reiki practitioners act as conduits for universal life force energy. Their mental and emotional state can influence the quality of the energy being channeled.
   - A clear and focused mind helps ensure that the energy transferred is pure and effective.

2. Client Sensitivity
   - Clients receiving Reiki are often in a heightened state of sensitivity and can pick up on the practitioner's energy. A balanced and centered practitioner can provide a more calming and healing experience.

Strategies for Practitioners to Manage Their Mind and Personal Issues

1. Self-Care and Regular Reiki Practice
   - Daily Self-Reiki: Practicing self-Reiki daily helps maintain the practitioner's own energy balance and mental clarity.
   - Regular Sessions with Other Practitioners: Receiving Reiki from other practitioners can provide additional support and healing for the practitioner's personal issues.
2. Mindfulness and Meditation
   - Meditation Practice: Regular meditation helps calm the mind, increase self-awareness, and manage stress.
   - Mindfulness Techniques: Practicing mindfulness throughout the day can help practitioners stay present and focused during sessions.
3. Setting Clear Intentions
   - Before each session, practitioners should set clear intentions to focus solely on the client's healing. This helps create a boundary between their issues and the Reiki session.

- Example Intention: "I set aside my personal concerns to focus fully on the healing needs of my client."
4. Grounding Techniques
   - Grounding exercises such as deep breathing, visualizing roots growing from the feet into the earth, or physical activities like walking can help practitioners stay centered and balanced.
5. Energy Cleansing
   - Clearing the Space: Smudging with sage, using sound (e.g., bells or singing bowls), or visualizing a white light cleansing the room can help clear negative energies from space.
   - Personal Energy Cleansing: Taking salt baths, using crystals, or performing energy-sweeping techniques can help clear the practitioner's energy field.
6. Journaling and Reflection
   - Keeping a journal to reflect on personal feelings and experiences can help practitioners process their emotions and gain insights.
   - Regular reflection on their practice and personal growth can aid in maintaining a balanced state of mind.
7. Professional Support
   - Practitioners should not hesitate to seek professional support if needed. Therapists, counselors, or spiritual advisors can guide and support personal issues.
8. Healthy Lifestyle Choices
   - Maintaining a healthy diet, regular exercise, and adequate sleep are essential for overall well-being and mental clarity.

- Avoiding substances that can cloud the mind, such as excessive alcohol or drugs, is also crucial.

Preparing for a Reiki Session

1. Pre-Session Rituals
   - Practitioners should engage in a pre-session ritual that includes grounding, setting intentions, and briefly meditating to center themselves.
   - Cleansing the energy in the room and around their body can also be part of the ritual.
2. During the Session
   - Practitioners should remain mindful and present throughout the session, continuously focusing on the flow of Reiki energy and the client's needs.
   - If personal thoughts or emotions arise, practitioners should acknowledge them without attachment and gently return their focus to the Reiki session.
3. Post-Session Self-Care
   - After a session, practitioners should take time to ground themselves, cleanse their energy, and reflect on the experience.
   - Engaging in a brief self-Reiki session or meditation can help reset their energy and prepare for the next session or the rest of their day.

Managing your own mind and personal issues is vital for Reiki practitioners to provide effective mental and emotional healing sessions. By practicing self-care, mindfulness, grounding, and energy cleansing, practitioners can ensure they remain balanced and centered, allowing them to channel Reiki energy more effectively. Regular reflection and professional support can also aid in addressing any personal issues, ensuring that practitioners maintain a clear and focused mind during their healing work.

Mental Healing

Reiki is a holistic healing technique that addresses well-being's physical, emotional, mental, and spiritual aspects. Mental healing through Reiki focuses on alleviating stress, anxiety, negative thought patterns, and other mental disturbances to promote clarity, peace, and mental well-being. Here's a detailed guide on how Reiki can assist in mental healing.

The Reiki Symbol for "Mental Healing" connects you directly with the receiver's Higher Self and Subconscious. "Mental Healing" can help transform misdirected energy so the receiver can experience optimism, love, and happiness. They can gain more awareness of past conditioning and programming. This is the first step toward healing. Fear, addictions, and other mental or spiritual disturbances can be influenced in a positive way. Inner strength and mental clarity will be attained. Fear and anger become trust, love, and total connection with the Self. Depression and guilt turn to the enjoyment of life, vitality, and courage.

Universal life energy helps you transform feelings with lower frequencies into those with higher frequencies.

Understanding Mental Healing with Reiki

1. Mind and Energy Connection
    *   The mind and body are interconnected; mental stress or disturbances can manifest as physical ailments. Reiki helps by balancing the body's energy flow, which promotes mental clarity and reduces psychological stress.

- Mental blockages can create disruptions in the body's energy field, leading to anxiety, depression, and other mental health issues. Reiki clears these blockages, facilitating mental healing.

2. Chakras and Mental Health
   - Chakras are energy centers in the body, each associated with different physical, emotional, and mental health aspects. Key chakras related to mental healing include:
     a. Crown Chakra (Sahasrara): Associated with higher consciousness, wisdom, and spiritual connection. Imbalances can lead to confusion and disconnection.
     b. Third Eye Chakra (Ajna): Linked to intuition, insight, and mental clarity. Imbalances can cause a lack of focus and mental fog.
     c. Throat Chakra (Vishuddha): Related to communication and truth. Imbalances can result in difficulties in expressing thoughts and emotions.

Reiki Symbols for Mental Healing

- Cho Ku Rei (Cho-Koo-Ray): Known as the power symbol, it helps ground and amplify healing energy.
- Sei He Ki (Say-Hey-Key): Specifically used for mental and emotional healing, it aids in balancing and harmonizing the mind.

In "Mental Healing," you can work with affirmations that describe a positive state you wish for yourself or with affirmations your client wishes for themselves.

Affirmations and Intentions

1. Setting clear intentions or affirmations before and during Reiki can enhance mental healing. Examples include "I release all mental stress" or "I welcome mental clarity and peace."
2. Combining Reiki with positive affirmations can reprogram the mind and replace negative thought patterns with positive ones.

Affirmations like the following may be used:

1. "I (name) love myself simply because I am as I am."
   This opens your heart, and the burden of fighting and rejecting yourself may dissolve gently.
2. "I (name) now love and accept my body."
   This is for physical healing.
3. "I (name) open my heart and now accept all my feelings."
   This is for emotional healing.
4. "My mental clarity is getting clearer every day."
   This is for mental healing.
5. "My meditations are getting deeper every day."
   This is for spiritual healing.

Benefits of Reiki Mental Healing

1. Stress Reduction
   - Reiki induces a state of deep relaxation, which helps reduce stress and anxiety. This calm state allows the mind to heal and rejuvenate.
2. Improved Focus and Clarity
   - Reiki enhances focus, concentration, and mental clarity by clearing mental blockages. It helps organize thoughts and make better decisions.
3. Emotional Balance
   - Reiki balances the mind and emotions, reducing mood swings, irritability, and mental turmoil. This balance promotes a sense of inner peace and stability.
4. Alleviation of Anxiety and Depression
   - Regular Reiki sessions can significantly reduce symptoms of anxiety and depression by addressing the root causes and clearing mental blockages.
5. Enhanced Intuition and Insight
   - By balancing the third eye chakra, Reiki enhances intuition and insight. This heightened awareness helps one understand oneself and one's surroundings better.
6. Better Sleep
   - Mental stress often leads to sleep disturbances. Reiki promotes relaxation and mental calmness, improving sleep quality and patterns.

Mental Healing Session:

"You must have the client's permission to do this healing, and your mind must be clear and empty of mental clutter so the session can be effective."

The session takes about 15 minutes and can be incorporated into a normal Reiki treatment.

1. Have the client sit on a chair.
2. Call upon your client's Higher Self and Healing Guide and your Higher Self and Reiki Master in Spirit to help you heal.
3. Place one hand on top of the Crown (7th) Chakra and the other across the occipital ridge, perpendicular to the first hand. Then, gently touching the Crown after each symbol, draw the RAKU, CHOKUREI, and SEHEKI symbols over the Crown Chakra.
4. Repeat the affirmation that describes the positive state you (or your client) wish for at this time.
5. To seal in the energy, draw the symbols over the Crown again, then either continue with a normal Reiki session or close the session in the same manner a normal Reiki session is closed.

Emotional Healing

Reiki is a holistic healing technique that works on the physical, mental, emotional, and spiritual levels. Emotional healing through Reiki focuses on addressing and releasing emotional blockages, trauma, and negative patterns that can impact a person's well-being. Here's everything you need to know about how Reiki can aid emotional healing.

Understanding Emotional Healing with Reiki

1. Energy Imbalance and Emotional Health
    *   Emotions are energy; like all energy, they must flow freely. When emotions are suppressed or unresolved, they create blockages in the body's energy field. These blockages can lead to emotional distress, mental health issues, and even physical ailments.
    *   Reiki helps to clear these blockages, restoring the natural flow of energy and promoting emotional balance and well-being.
2. Chakras and Emotional Healing
    *   Chakras are energy centers in the body that correspond to different aspects of physical, emotional, and spiritual health. Emotional healing in Reiki often involves balancing the chakras, particularly:
        a. Heart Chakra (Anahata): Associated with love, compassion, and forgiveness.
        b. Solar Plexus Chakra (Manipura): Linked to self-esteem, power, and identity.

    c. Sacral Chakra (Svadhisthana): Connected to emotions, relationships, and creativity.
- By harmonizing these chakras, Reiki helps release emotional pain and promotes feelings of peace and happiness.

Reiki Symbols for Emotional Healing

Sei He Ki (Say-Hey-Key): The primary symbol used in Reiki for emotional healing. It helps balance emotions, clear mental blockages, and promote harmony and peace.

Benefits of Reiki Emotional Healing

1. Stress Reduction and Relaxation
   - Reiki induces a state of deep relaxation, which helps reduce stress and anxiety. This calm state allows the mind and body to heal more effectively.
2. Release of Emotional Blockages
   - By clearing blocked energy, Reiki helps release suppressed emotions and unresolved trauma. This release can lead to profound emotional and mental relief.
3. Enhanced Emotional Awareness
   - Reiki enhances self-awareness, helping individuals recognize and understand their emotions better. This awareness is the first step toward healing and personal growth.
4. Improved Relationships
   - As individuals heal emotionally, they often find that their relationships improve. They

become more compassionate, understanding, and capable of healthy communication.

5. Greater Emotional Resilience
   - Regular Reiki sessions can build emotional resilience, helping individuals cope better with life's challenges and stresses.
6. Spiritual Growth
   - Emotional healing through Reiki often leads to spiritual growth. As individuals release emotional baggage, they may feel more connected to their higher self and the universe.

Reiki emotional healing is a gentle yet powerful method for addressing and releasing emotional pain and trauma. Reiki helps balance emotions, reduce stress, and promote overall well-being by restoring the natural flow of energy in the body. Whether through regular sessions with a practitioner or self-Reiki practices, integrating Reiki into your life can lead to profound emotional and spiritual growth.

Procedure:

1. Have the client sit or lie down.
2. Get a chair for yourself.
3. Place one hand on the client's brow chakra and the other on the occipital ridge (back of their neck).
4. Call upon your client's higher self, healing guide, and your Reiki Master in Spirit to help you heal.
5. Bring in the appropriate symbol (Sei He Ki).
6. This is the only position where you can trade hands if you need to. A session can last up to one hour.
7. When the session is completed, thank the guides and · Reiki master for their help.

Reiki In Daily Life

Children and Reiki:

Reiki treatments on children are the same as for adults, except they take less time since they are smaller and require fewer hand positions.

Children can be attuned to 1st-degree Reiki at any age because it deals with the physical body. Children should understand emotions and have mental clarity before they are attuned to a 2nd Degree. They should have a concept of spirituality before being attuned to a Master's Degree Reiki.

Reiki on Plants and Animals:

Plants and trees love Reiki energy. They respond by revealing strong and hearty growth, good blossom development, and a long life.

Most animals accept Reiki energy. Treat all mammals in the same manner that you would a person. Birds have a very sensitive system, so always emphasize the importance of bringing through the highest Reiki energy so they can easily use it.

Reiki First Aid

- *Broken Bones:* DO NOT DO BEFOE THE BONE IS SET!!! After a Doctor sets the fracture, you can lay your hands directly on the cast to help it heal.
- *Bruising:* Give Reiki immediately and directly on the bruise for 20 to 30 minutes.

- *Burns:* Give 20 to 30 minutes of Reiki just above the burned skin. Blisters are less likely to appear if you can give it right away.
- *Fear:* Lay your hands on the Solar Plexus (3rd) Chakra and the back of the head and do a mental healing.
- *Insect Bites:* If you can give Reiki immediately, for 20 to 30 minutes, you may be able to keep the swelling down.
- *Shock/Accident:* While waiting for a Doctor, give Reiki to the Solar Plexus (3rd) Chakra and the Root (1st) Chakra. Then, apply Reiki energy to their shoulders.
  Sprains: Give Reiki energy to the sprained area for 30 to 60 minutes. Repeat several times depending on the severity of the sprain.

Reiki Level 2 – Practitioner Homework

1) Why would you use the Reiki symbols?

_____
_____
_____
_____
_____

2) What is the primary learning objective in level 2 Reiki?

_____
_____
_____
_____
_____
_____

3) Describe your first Reiki treatment on a client (Friend or Family).

_____
_____
_____
_____
_____
_____
_____
_____
_____
_____
_____

Reiki Level 2 – Client Case Study Example

HEALTH FORM

Date: _____

Clients Name: _____

Phone Number: _____

E-mail: _____

Address:_____

City: _____

Postal Code _____

Birth date (Month): _____

Practitioner (you): _____

QUESTIONS TO ASK:

How are you feeling today?

_____

In your opinion, are you stressed?

_____

Are you undergoing any other therapies?

_____

Any other health or area of concern?

_____

What are your expectations for this session?

_____

Have you had this type or similar session before? No / Yes

Client signature: (acknowledgment and permission of session) _____

FINDINGS / ISSUES: *(mark down)*

Front   Back

Physical:

_____
_____

Mental:

_____
_____

Emotional:

_____
_____

Spiritual:

_____
_____

Opening Your Own Reiki Clinic: The Basics

Starting a Reiki clinic can be a fulfilling way to share your healing practice with others. Here are the essential steps and rules to consider when opening your own Reiki clinic, whether you plan to charge for your services or not.

If Not Charging Any Money

1. Personal Liability Insurance
   - Obtain personal liability insurance to protect yourself in case of any claims or accidents during your sessions. This is essential for safeguarding your practice.
2. Client Forms
   - Ensure that you fill out a client form for each session. This form should include the client's personal information, health history, and consent for treatment. Keeping detailed records is essential for both legal and practical reasons.

If Charging Money

1. Legal Company Name
   - Register a legal company name for your Reiki clinic. This formalizes your business and is

often required for various legal and financial transactions.

2. GST Number
   - Canada: If your annual income exceeds $30,000, you must register for a GST (Goods and Services Tax) number. This allows you to charge and remit GST on your services.
3. Personal Liability Insurance
   - Just as with non-paid services, having personal liability insurance is crucial. This protects you against potential claims or accidents during your practice.
4. Client Forms
   - Fill out a client form for each session detailing the client's personal information, health history, and consent. Maintaining these records is crucial for compliance and effective practice management. Ten years
5. Receipts
   - Provide a receipt for each session. This keeps your clients informed and helps you maintain accurate financial records.
6. Business Taxes
   - Keep track of your income and expenses throughout the year, and ensure you pay your business taxes at the end of the year. Consult an accountant to understand your tax obligations and ensure compliance with all relevant laws.

Additional Tips for Success

7. Location:
    - Choose a comfortable, accessible location for your clinic. Ensure that the space is serene and conducive to healing, with appropriate privacy for your clients.
8. Marketing
    - Promote your clinic through various channels such as social media, local community boards, and word of mouth. Offering introductory sessions or workshops can help attract new clients.
9. Professional Development
    - Continue to enhance your skills and knowledge through ongoing education and training. Staying updated with the latest in Reiki and complementary therapies can enhance your practice and attract more clients.
10. Networking
    - Connect with other holistic health practitioners and local wellness centers. Networking can provide referral opportunities and support your business growth.
11. Client Communication
    - Maintain clear and compassionate communication with your clients. Understanding their needs and providing tailored sessions can enhance their experience and promote positive word-of-mouth referrals.

12. Compliance and Ethics
- Adhere to all local regulations and ethical guidelines in your practice. This includes respecting client confidentiality, obtaining informed consent, and providing professional and compassionate care.

By following these guidelines and focusing on professional integrity and client care, you can successfully open and operate your own Reiki clinic.

REIKI LEVEL 3 – MASTER

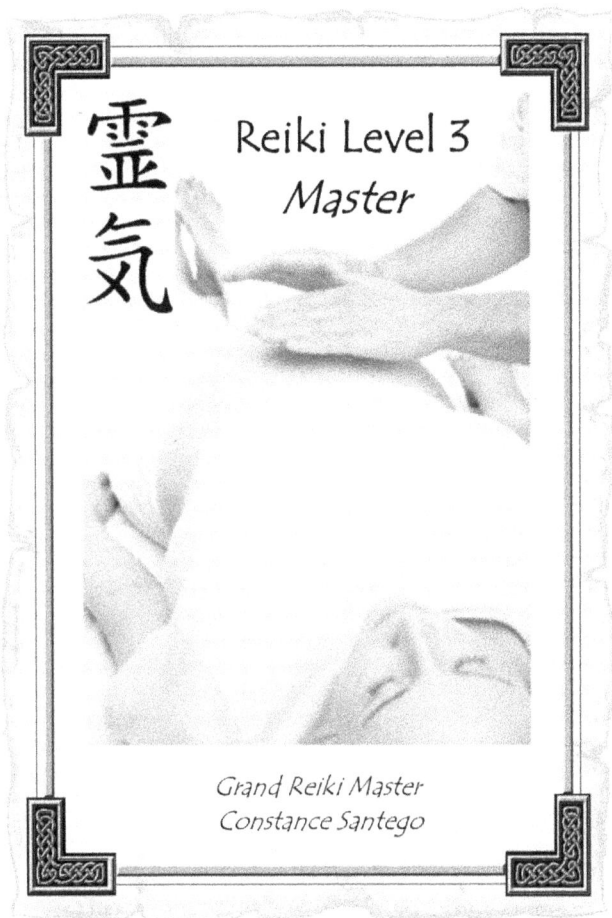

Reiki Level 3
Master

霊気

Grand Reiki Master
Constance Santego

Level 3: Shinpiden

Shinpiden, meaning "Mystery Teachings" or "Master Teachings," is the advanced level of Reiki training. It focuses on mastery of Reiki energy, spiritual growth, and the ability to teach and attune others.

Reiki Level 3 Lesson Plan

2, 3-hour live classes

1st class

- Talk about spiritual healing

2nd part of 1st class
Listen and Subscribe

> https://youtu.be/4F-re1mkiCk

or *Read* the "Apprentice" Meditation

  o Draw the level 3 symbol on each student
  o Finish meditation
- Have each student talk about what they experienced

2nd class

- Talk about teaching Reiki
- Try all the spiritual Reiki hands-on techniques.

Reiki Spiritual Healing

Reiki spiritual healing focuses on balancing and harmonizing the spiritual aspects of an individual. It helps connect with higher consciousness, enhance spiritual awareness, and align with one's true self. This form of healing is integral to holistic well-being, addressing the physical and emotional bodies and the spiritual body.

Key Concepts in Reiki Spiritual Healing

1. **Universal Life Force Energy**
    *   Reiki is based on universal life force energy flowing through all living things. This energy is believed to be spiritually guided and can be channeled by a Reiki practitioner to promote healing.
2. **Spiritual Connection**
    *   Reiki helps individuals connect with their higher self and spiritual guides. This connection can provide guidance, insight, and a deeper understanding of one's life purpose.
3. **Chakras and Spiritual Healing**
    *   The chakra system plays a crucial role in spiritual healing. Each chakra is associated with different aspects of spiritual development and consciousness. Balancing the chakras can enhance spiritual growth and enlightenment.

Master Symbols

Raku: Is one of the lesser-known but very powerful symbols in Reiki, particularly associated with the attunement process. It is not commonly used in regular Reiki sessions but plays a crucial role during the attunements in the Master level of Reiki training.

Dai Ko Myo: The master symbol in Reiki, representing enlightenment and spiritual empowerment. It is used to open up higher levels of spiritual awareness and connection.

Benefits of Reiki Spiritual Healing

1. Enhanced Spiritual Awareness
    *   Reiki helps individuals become more aware of their spiritual nature and connection to the universe. This awareness can lead to a deeper sense of purpose and fulfillment.
2. Alignment with Higher Self
    *   By balancing the spiritual body, Reiki helps align individuals with their higher self, promoting inner peace and harmony.
3. Clearing Spiritual Blockages
    *   Reiki can help clear blockages in the spiritual body, allowing for a smoother flow of energy and a stronger connection to spiritual guides and higher consciousness.
4. Increased Intuition and Insight
    *   Regular Reiki sessions can enhance intuitive abilities and provide deeper insights into personal and spiritual matters.

5. Emotional and Mental Clarity
   - Spiritual healing often leads to greater emotional and mental clarity, as it addresses the root causes of emotional and mental imbalances from a spiritual perspective.

Reiki spiritual healing is a profound and transformative practice that addresses the spiritual aspects of an individual's being. By balancing and harmonizing the spiritual body, Reiki helps individuals connect with their higher self, gain deeper spiritual insights, and align with their true purpose. Practitioners play a vital role in facilitating this process, and by maintaining their spiritual practices, they can provide effective and meaningful healing to their clients. Integrating spiritual healing into daily life can lead to lasting benefits and a deeper sense of spiritual fulfillment.

LEVEL 3 MEDITATION FOR ATTUNEMENT

Part "One" Of Level 3 Attunement Meditation

You have a choice:

1) Listen to the level 3 meditation on YouTube https://youtu.be/4F-re1mkiCk

Or

2) In class:
   a. Read the 1st part of the meditation,
   b. Draw the reiki symbols on each student's crown, heart chakras, and both palms. *(by holding Hui Yin and taking a Kidney Breath),*
   c. Read 2nd part of the meditation,
   d. Water Ritual (Draw the Symbols over the lemon water),
   e. Say the Raku Kei Affirmation

Journey Into Mastery

Note: This is a very advanced meditation! I use it only after two weeks of causal plane work with my students before giving them this meditation to prepare them for this release. Until you are experienced with causal plane work, I encourage you to design a much less intense clearing exercise for your students. For example, you could use a body Chakra clearing where all the old stagnate energy from each Chakra is blown out into a bubble, then dissolved into neutralized energy and sent down into the energy recycling center in the center of the Earth. Each Chakra could then be filled with Reiki energy.

Read This Meditation

"I'm now going to be taking you on a journey into Mastery. It doesn't matter whether you see, feel, hear, or simply know it's happening. The most important thing that you can do for yourself is simply allow yourself to be ready to release now.

Bring your awareness to your first light body center... your Root Chakra, which represents survival, manifestation, and material gain. Allow your Reiki Master to assist you in removing all the blockages.....Allowing the release of any stuck energy around money, material gain, physical challenges, pain, or physical abuse. Anytime your needs were not met at a survival level, let all of those blockages go now. Any past lives where survival was a struggle....Remove all the blockages in this lifetime or past lifetimes. You don't need them anymore...... And now, allow your Reiki Master in Spirit to assist you in filling the survival light body center back up.... Healing it, harmonizing and balancing it....Knowing that you are unlimited in your ability to earn a living while pursuing your purpose....Knowing that you are unlimited in your ability to have a strong, healthy body that you love and that works perfectly for you....Knowing that you are unlimited in your ability to create your survival in a healthy, harmonious, positive, prosperous way.

Now bring your attention to your second light body center...your Spleen Chakra....your sexual and creativity center....And allow your Reiki Master in Spirit to assist you in removing any blockages.....Anytime you were judged for your sexual feelings.....Anytime you were abused.... All the fears of intimacy....let them go now. Anytime somebody judged your creativity....And now past lives... All the blockages around your sexuality and creativity.....Let them all go.....Now allow your Reiki Master in Spirit to assist you in filling up your second light body center..........healing it, harmonizing it and balancing it....Knowing that you are unlimited in your ability to honor yourself as a sensual being and to draw loving, nurturing, supportive, sensual experiences to yourself in a perfect and harmonious way for you.....Knowing that you are unlimited in your ability to utilize your creativity in any form you choose.

Now, moving your awareness up to your third light body center, Your will, your willpower, and your emotional center....And now allowing your Reiki Master to assist you in removing all the blockages....Anytime that you felt like a victim... Anytime you felt like you had no choice....Anytime you did anything that you did not want to do....Release all fears now... All fears of being hurt... on body, mind, spirit, and emotional levels.... Releasing all anger....any jealousy....all the guilt you ever had....Karma ends when you forgive yourself. Forgive yourself now and move on. Anytime you were emotionally abused.... And now, past lives where you abused your power....Past lives where you allowed others to abuse you......Release all the blockages now.....Blockages surrounding your will, your will power and your yourself to have this experience. I'd like you now to imagine your soul's energy in your Root Chakra at the base of your spine. Now imagine pulling your soul's energy up through your Root Chakra, all the way up to your Crown Chakra, at the top of

your head. Feel it as it goes through your Spleen.....through your Solar Plexus.....through your Heart Chakra.........through your Throat.....through your 3rd Eye Chakra..... And feel it as it enters your Crown Chakra at the top of your head......
Now, I want you to imagine a ladder of enlightenment, a golden ladder that goes all the way out to the enlightenment plane. I'd like you now to imagine yourself beginning to climb this ladder....climbing up out of your body, out through the ceiling, out through the roof of this building....Now look around. How far can you see?.....Continue climbing until you're a mile above the city. Now what can you see?....As you continue to climb, I'm going to count from one to three and when I get to three, you're going to be half way between the Earth and the Moon climbing your ladder of enlightenment. One....your soul already knows exactly where that spot is. Two....it's just a matter of allowing yourself to get there.

Three....there you are....halfway between the Earth and the Moon. Looking down at the Earth what can you see?....Looking up at the Moon now I want you to climb higher and higher. We're going to climb your ladder of enlightenment all the way past the Moon....All the way out to the enlightenment plane. I'm going to count from one to three again, and when I get to three, you will be climbing up off your ladder onto the enlightenment plane. One....your soul knows exactly where the enlightenment plane is. Two....it's just a matter of allowing yourself to be led there. Three....there you are, climbing up off your ladder, onto the enlightenment plane.... You will notice the light is very bright and vivid. You can feel the unconditional love that permeates and penetrates everything. You may hear songs, melodies, harps.... And you know that this is a place of infinite peace, joy, love, harmony, and enlightenment.....Now, I'd like you to call upon your Reiki Master in Spirit to join you here.....And I'd like you to ask it to assist you in removing all the blockages, barriers, fears, limitations, or old, outdated patterns emotions........Let them all go.....And now, allowing your Reiki Master to assist you in filling this center up....healing it, harmonizing it, and balancing it....Knowing that you are unlimited in your ability to manifest with ease....Knowing that you are unlimited in your ability to be self-empowered and to make the decisions and the choices that are for your highest good all of the time.....Knowing that you are unlimited in your ability to experience peace, love, joy, bliss, harmony and true intimacy.

And now moving your awareness up to your fourth light body center, your Heart Chakra....And allowing your Reiki Master to assist you in removing all of the blockages surrounding your love and affinity, which means unconditional love for yourself and others........Anytime you were judged for any reason........Anytime you judged somebody else....Anytime you felt hurt on a heart level.....All the conditional love that you ever experienced for any reason....Let them all go now, ...all of the blockages.... And now past lives... Anytime that your heart was broken, past or present...consciously or unconsciously....Release all the blockages surrounding your love and affinity for yourself and others, past or present, this lifetime or past lifetimes....Let it all go.....And now, allow your Reiki Master to assist you in filling this light body center back up... healing it, harmonizing it and balancing it... Knowing that you are unlimited in your ability to love yourself and others in a healthy, appropriate way...Knowing that you are unlimited in your ability to draw healthy, nurturing, supportive, loving relationships to you and to know that you deserve them.

Now, moving your awareness up to your fifth light body center...your Throat Chakra... your communication center....And allowing the release of all the blockages surrounding your communication and your intelligence....Anytime you were talking, and nobody listened to you... Anytime you felt unheard....Anytime you felt misunderstood....Anytime you hid your intellect....Anytime you said somebody's truth instead of your own....Anytime you didn't speak your own truth....Let all of the blockages go now....And now all of the blockages from past lifetimes regarding your communication and intellect....Anytime your communication or lack of it, got you into trouble....past or present....Now allow your Reiki Master to assist you in removing all of the blockages surrounding your communication and intellect, conscious or unconscious, past or present... Let it go.....And now allow your Reiki Master to assist you in filling this center back up...healing it, harmonizing it, balancing it... Knowing that you are unlimited in your ability to speak your truth in perfect form and with perfect content....Knowing that you are unlimited in your ability to use your intellect in ways that serve you best.

And now, move your awareness up to your sixth light body center, your Third Eye, your psychic and perception center. Allowing your Reiki Master to assist you in removing all blockages surrounding your perception of things....Anytime you were judged for not seeing something... Anytime you judged yourself for being in denial....Anytime you tried to hide the truth from yourself....Anytime somebody judged your intuition or psychic abilities.....Anytime you didn't trust your own psychic abilities....Past lives where you ignored your perception of things....Past lives where you ignored your healing abilities or your psychic abilities.....Release all the blockages now... surrounding your perception, psychic abilities, healing abilities, conscious or unconscious, past lives or present...Let them all go...And now, allowing your Reiki Master to assist you in filling this center back up, healing it, harmonizing it and balancing it...........Knowing that you are unlimited in your ability to have clear, accurate perception and to act on it.....Knowing that you are unlimited in your ability to utilize your intuition, your psychic ability, your sixth sense and trusting it implicitly....Knowing that you are unlimited in your ability to use your unlimited healing abilities....Allow yourself to have it....Allow yourself to honor it.

And now, moving your awareness up to your seventh light body center........your Crown Chakra.... your spiritual center....Allowing your Reiki Master to assist you in removing any blockages surrounding your spirituality or your religious beliefs....Anytime you were judged for your spiritual or religious beliefs....Anytime you felt abandoned by God or your higher self....Anytime you abandoned God or your higher self....Release it now...all the blockages....And now, in past lives where you had to hide your spiritual truth....let it go now... you don't have to be limited anymore....Release all of the blockages surrounding your spiritual or religious beliefs, conscious or unconscious.....Allowing your Reiki Master to assist you in filling this light body center back up, healing it, harmonizing it and balancing it.....Knowing that you are unlimited in your ability to be at one with your higher self....Knowing that you are unlimited in your ability to connect with, be supported by, and be one with your Source or God....Knowing that you are limitless in living your spiritual truth, whatever that may be....Knowing that the universe will support you in that.....Knowing that your higher self...guardian angel....the divine Source... God, in whatever form you perceive it in, always supports, nurtures, and loves you unconditionally.

Attune the Student:

1. While the student holds their "Hui Yin," open their crown chakra with the Raku Symbol, then draw the Reiki Level 3- Raku symbol into their crown, heart, and palms.
2. Now, the student takes a "Kidney Breath."
3. Close their crown with the Raku symbol...
4. Then, continue the second part of the meditation...

Reiki Level 3 Symbol

Reiki "Master" Symbols

Raku

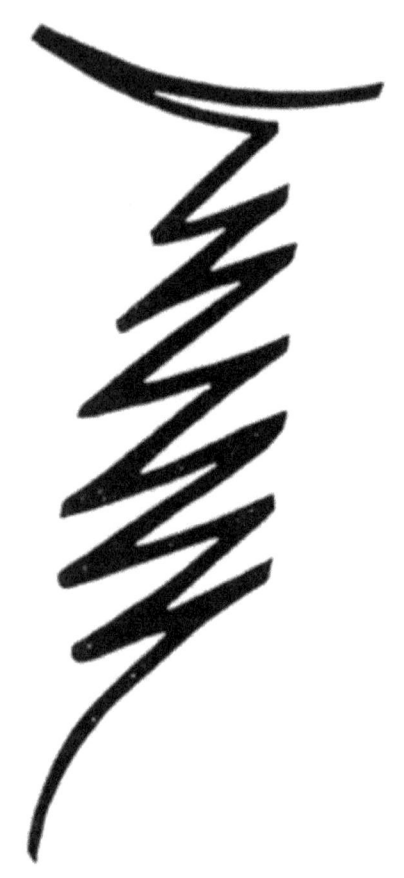

The Raku symbol is one of the lesser-known but very powerful symbols in Reiki, particularly associated with the attunement process. It is not commonly used in regular Reiki sessions but plays a crucial role during the attunements in the Master level of Reiki training.

Overview of the Raku Symbol

1. Appearance
   - The Raku symbol is typically drawn as a zigzag or lightning bolt shape. It is simple in form but carries a deep and powerful energy.
2. Meaning and Purpose
   - Separation and Grounding: The primary purpose of the Raku symbol is to separate the energies of the Reiki Master and the student after an attunement. It grounds the energies and helps in sealing the attunement process.
   - Energy Release: Raku is also used to release negative energy and blockages from the body, allowing the individual to be more receptive to healing.
   - Balancing: It aids in balancing and stabilizing the energy within the recipient's body, ensuring that the newly attuned energies are properly integrated.

Using the Raku Symbol

1. During Attunements
   - Final Step in Attunement: Raku is typically used at the end of the attunement process. The Reiki Master draws the symbol down the

student's spine to help ground and seal the energies.

- Grounding Energy: By drawing the Raku symbol, the Master ensures that the student's energy is grounded, helping to prevent energy overload and ensuring the smooth flow of Reiki energy.

2. Clearing and Grounding
    - Energy Clearing: Although less common, Raku can be used during a Reiki session to help clear the energy field and ground the recipient. This can be particularly useful for individuals who feel ungrounded or are experiencing significant energetic blockages.
    - Personal Use: Reiki Masters may use Raku on themselves to ground their energy after a session or attunement, helping to release any residual energy picked up from the recipient.
3. If the area is smaller than a walnut, do not use the Chokurei.

Steps to Draw and Use Raku

1. Visualize the Symbol
    - Before drawing Raku, take a moment to visualize the symbol in your mind. See it as a powerful lightning bolt filled with grounding energy.
2. Drawing Raku
    - Start at the top and draw a zigzag pattern downwards. The number of zigzag lines can vary, but the most important aspect is the intention behind the drawing.

- As you draw, focus on the intention of grounding, sealing, and balancing the energy.

3. Grounding the Energy
   - Draw Raku from the top of the head down the recipient's spine. Visualize the symbol's energy grounding deeply into the Earth.
   - If using it for personal grounding, draw the symbol down your own body, either physically with your hand or mentally with your mind's eye.

4. Sealing the Attunement
   - After completing the attunement process, draw Raku to seal the energies within the student. This helps integrate the new energies and ensures they remain balanced and grounded.

Practical Tips for Using Raku

Clear Intentions

1. Always set a clear intention before using the Raku symbol. Whether you are grounding, clearing, or sealing, your intention will direct the energy effectively.
   - Example Intention: "I use the power of Raku to ground and stabilize the energies, ensuring balance and harmony."

2. Practice Regularly
   - Practice drawing the Raku symbol regularly to become familiar with its energy and form. This will help you use it more effectively during attunements and healing sessions.

3. Ground Yourself

- Ensure you are well-grounded before using Raku on others. Grounding yourself will help you channel the symbol's energy more effectively and prevent energy overload.

4. Combine with Other Symbols
   - Raku can be combined with other Reiki symbols, such as Cho Ku Rei and Sei He Ki, to enhance its effects. For example, Cho Ku Rei is used for power, Sei He Ki is used for emotional balance, and Raku is used for grounding and sealing.

Benefits of the Raku Symbol

1. Enhanced Grounding
   - It helps practitioners and recipients feel more grounded and connected to the Earth, providing stability and balance.
2. Energy Integration
   - Facilitates the integration of new energies during attunements, ensuring they are properly absorbed and balanced within the recipient's body.
3. Energy Clearing
   - Effective in releasing negative energies and blockages, promoting a clearer and more balanced energy flow.
4. Sealing and Protection
   - It seals the energy within the recipient, protecting it from external influences and ensuring it remains stable and harmonious.

The Raku Reiki symbol is a powerful tool primarily used during attunements to ground and seal energies. While it is not commonly used in everyday Reiki sessions, its role in the attunement process is vital for ensuring the proper integration and balance of new energies. By understanding and practicing the use of Raku, Reiki practitioners can enhance their ability to provide effective and grounded healing to their students and clients.

Raku Affirmation

" I believe there is a great cosmic magnet that manifests as the spirit of truth, love, and light. This cosmic magnet lives in me as part of my divine nature.

I recognize the pure white light in my soul. This holy spirit in my soul continually guides me in everything I think, say, and do.

Through my magnetic personality, I pour my resources into the world. As I give, so shall I receive, living my life happily, expressing creatively, and experiencing perfect well-being.

So be it now and forever".

Dai Ko Myo

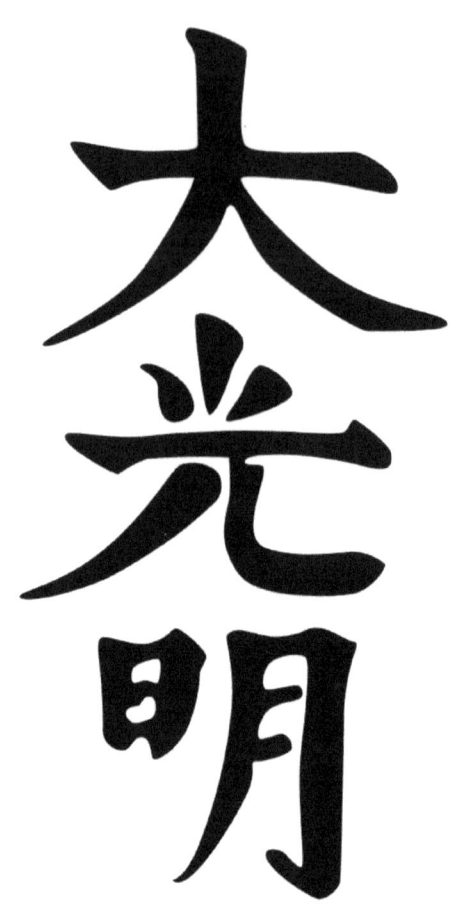

The Dai Ko Myo symbol is one of the most important and powerful symbols in Reiki, often referred to as the Master Symbol. It is primarily used by Reiki Masters and is introduced during the third level of Reiki training (Reiki Master level). This symbol encompasses the energy of all the other Reiki symbols and represents the highest level of spiritual enlightenment and empowerment.

Overview of the Dai Ko Myo Symbol

2) Appearance
   a. The Dai Ko Myo symbol has a complex design, often depicted as a series of spirals and lines. The exact form can vary slightly between different Reiki traditions, but its core essence remains the same.
3) Meaning and Purpose
   a. Enlightenment and Empowerment: Dai Ko Myo means "Great Shining Light" or "Great Enlightenment." It is used to enhance spiritual growth and personal empowerment.
   b. Healing at All Levels: This symbol is believed to work on all levels – physical, emotional, mental, and spiritual – providing comprehensive healing.
   c. Amplification of Energy: Dai Ko Myo amplifies the energy of other Reiki symbols and techniques, making it a powerful tool for deep healing.

Uses of the Dai Ko Myo Symbol

1. Attunements
   - Initiation: Dai Ko Myo is primarily used during the Reiki attunement process, which helps initiate and empower students. It opens up the student's energy channels to higher frequencies of Reiki energy.
   - Sealing the Energy: The symbol is used to seal the attunement, ensuring that the new energy pathways remain open and balanced.
2. Healing Sessions
   - Deep Healing: Practitioners use Dai Ko Myo for deep healing sessions, targeting the symptoms and root causes of ailments.
   - Spiritual Growth: It can be used to facilitate spiritual awakening and growth, helping individuals connect with their higher self and spiritual guides.
   - Energy Amplification: Dai Ko Myo can be combined with other Reiki symbols, such as Cho Ku Rei and Sei He Ki, to amplify their effects and provide more profound healing.
3. Self-Reiki
   - Personal Empowerment: Practitioners use this symbol on themselves to enhance their own spiritual development and personal empowerment.
   - Daily Practice: Incorporating Dai Ko Myo into daily self-Reiki practice helps maintain a high vibrational state and spiritual alignment.

How to Use the Dai Ko Myo Symbol

1. Drawing the Symbol
   - Visualize the Symbol: Start by visualizing the symbol in your mind's eye. Imagine it glowing with a bright, radiant light.
   - Drawing with Intention: Draw the symbol with your hand or visualize drawing it in your mind. Focus on the intention behind the symbol, whether it's for healing, empowerment, or spiritual growth.
2. Chanting and Meditating
   - Chanting the Name: Saying "Dai Ko Myo" out loud or silently in your mind can help activate the symbol's energy. Repeating the name several times can deepen the connection.
   - Meditation: Meditate on the symbol, visualizing it enveloping you or your client in its radiant light. This can enhance the healing process and facilitate spiritual insights.
3. Combining with Other Symbols
   - Cho Ku Rei: Use Dai Ko Myo with Cho Ku Rei to enhance the power and focus of the energy.
   - Sei He Ki: Combine with Sei He Ki for emotional and mental healing.
   - Hon Sha Ze Sho Nen: Use Hon Sha Ze Sho Nen for distant or past-life healing.

Benefits of the Dai Ko Myo Symbol

1. Enhanced Spiritual Growth
   - Helps individuals connect with their higher self, spiritual guides, and universal consciousness, promoting spiritual enlightenment and growth.
2. Comprehensive Healing
   - Works on all levels of the being – physical, emotional, mental, and spiritual – providing holistic healing.
3. Increased Energy Flow
   - Amplifies the flow of Reiki energy, making healing sessions more powerful and effective.
4. Protection and Cleansing
   - Provides protection against negative energies and helps cleanse the energy field of both the practitioner and the recipient.
5. Empowerment
   - Empowers practitioners, enhancing their ability to channel Reiki energy and perform effective healings.

Practical Tips for Using Dai Ko Myo

1. Clear Intentions
    - Always set a clear intention before using Dai Ko Myo. This directs the energy effectively and enhances the healing process.
    - Example Intention: "I use Dai Ko Myo to enhance spiritual growth and provide deep healing on all levels."
2. Practice Regularly
    - Incorporate the symbol into your daily Reiki practice to become more familiar and comfortable with its energy.
3. Ground Yourself
    - Ensure you are well-grounded before using the symbol to prevent energy overload and maintain a balanced flow.
4. Stay Open
    - Be open to the spiritual insights and guidance that may come through when using Dai Ko Myo. This symbol often facilitates deeper spiritual awareness and understanding.

The Dai Ko Myo symbol is a powerful and transformative tool in the Reiki Master's arsenal. Its primary purpose is to facilitate spiritual enlightenment and deep healing on all levels. By understanding and practicing the use of Dai Ko Myo, Reiki practitioners can enhance their healing abilities and support their clients' spiritual growth and well-being. Regular use of this symbol can lead to profound personal empowerment and a deeper connection to the universal life force energy.

White Light

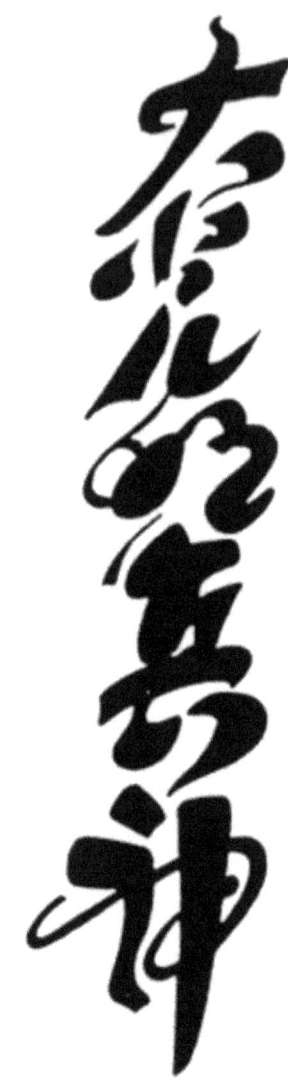

The Reiki White Light Symbol

The Reiki White Light Symbol, also known as the White Light or the Great White Light, is powerful and often revered in the practice of Reiki. While it is not one of the traditional Usui Reiki symbols, it is widely used in various Reiki traditions and healing practices. This symbol represents pure, divine energy and is associated with spiritual enlightenment, protection, and profound healing.

Overview of the Reiki White Light Symbol

a. Appearance
    a. The White Light Symbol has no specific drawn form, unlike traditional Reiki symbols. It is often visualized as a radiant white light or a beam of light descending from the heavens.
b. Meaning and Purpose
    a. Divine Energy: The White Light Symbol represents pure, unconditional love and divine energy from the highest spiritual realms.
    b. Spiritual Enlightenment is associated with spiritual awakening, enlightenment, and connecting with higher consciousness.
    c. Protection and Purification: The symbol is used for protection against negative energies and for purifying the mind, body, and spirit.

Uses of the Reiki White Light Symbol

1. Spiritual Healing
    • Connection to Higher Self: The White Light Symbol helps in connecting with the higher self

and spiritual guides. It opens channels to receive divine guidance and wisdom.
- Meditation: Practitioners use the symbol during meditation to enhance spiritual awareness and achieve a state of deep peace and enlightenment.

2. Protection
- Creating Protective Shields: Visualizing the White Light can create a protective shield around oneself or others, guarding against negative energies and influences.
- Space Clearing: It can be used to cleanse and protect physical spaces, ensuring they remain energetically pure and safe.

3. Healing Sessions
- Enhancing Reiki Energy: The White Light Symbol can be invoked during Reiki sessions to amplify the healing energy and bring in the highest vibrational frequencies.
- Aura Cleansing: It effectively cleans and strengthens the aura, removes blockages, and restores balance.

4. Distant Healing
- Sending Healing Energy: The symbol can be used in distant healing sessions to send powerful, high-frequency energy across time and space to those in need.

How to Use the Reiki White Light Symbol

1. Visualization Techniques
   - Meditation: During meditation, visualize a beam of radiant white light descending from above, enveloping you in pure energy. Imagine this light filling your entire being and connecting you with the divine.
   - Healing Sessions: While performing Reiki, visualize the White Light flowing through your hands and into the recipient, filling them with healing and protective energy.
2. Chanting and Affirmations
   - Chanting: Although the White Light Symbol does not have a specific name to chant, focusing on words like "Divine Light" or "Pure Light" can help activate its energy.
   - Affirmations: Use positive affirmations such as "I am surrounded by divine white light" or "The white light of purity fills and protects me."
3. Creating Protective Shields
   - Personal Protection: Visualize the White Light forming a shield around you, protecting you from any negative energies or influences.
   - Space Clearing: Envision the White Light filling and purifying a room or space, creating a sacred and protected environment.
4. Enhancing Other Reiki Symbols
   - Combination with Traditional Symbols: Use the White Light Symbol in conjunction with traditional Reiki symbols like Cho Ku Rei, Sei He Ki, and Dai Ko Myo to enhance their effects and bring in higher vibrational energy.

Benefits of the Reiki White Light Symbol

1. Spiritual Growth and Enlightenment
   - Helps in achieving a higher state of consciousness, spiritual awakening, and a deeper connection with the divine.
2. Powerful Healing Energy
   - Amplifies the effectiveness of Reiki healing sessions, bringing in pure and potent energy that promotes comprehensive healing.
3. Protection and Purification
   - Creates a protective shield against negative energies and purifies the mind, body, and spirit, ensuring a safe and positive healing environment.
4. Enhanced Intuition and Guidance
   - Facilitates clearer communication with spiritual guides and enhances intuitive abilities, providing guidance and wisdom.
   - Practical Tips for Using the Reiki White Light Symbol
5. Set Clear Intentions
   - Always set a clear intention when invoking the White Light Symbol. Your intention directs the energy effectively, whether for protection, healing, or spiritual growth.
6. Regular Practice
   - Incorporate the White Light Symbol into your regular Reiki practice and meditation sessions to familiarize yourself with its energy and effects.

7. Stay Grounded
   - While working with high-frequency energy like the White Light, ensure you stay grounded. This helps maintain balance and integrate energy smoothly.
8. Trust the Process
   - Trust in the power of the White Light Symbol and the divine energy it represents. Have faith in its ability to bring about profound healing and transformation.

The Reiki White Light Symbol is a powerful and versatile spiritual healing, protection, and enlightenment tool. While it is not part of the traditional Usui Reiki system, it is widely embraced in various Reiki practices for its profound benefits. Understanding and incorporating the White Light Symbol into your Reiki practice can enhance your healing abilities, achieve spiritual growth, and create a safe and protected environment for yourself and others.

Part "Two" Of Level 3 Attunement Meditation

Read this second part after drawing the symbols:

Now, you're going to notice a doorway....On the other side of this doorway, on the enlightenment plane are all of the other true masters of the universe waiting to meet you.....I want you now to go up to this doorway....Before we go through it, I want you to allow your Reiki Master to assist you in removing anything else that would stop you from being the Master that you are.....On the other side of this doorway is unconditional love for you. Anything that is not love cannot go through this door..... Any fears, judgments, blockages, barriers, lies, untruths, or denials aren't love. Allow your Reiki Master to take all the rest of the blockages, barriers, fears, limitations, and old outdated patterns from anywhere within you on a soul level and on a body level and release them now.....And now walk through the doorway...and be absorbed, be filled, be embraced with unconditional love in all aspects of your life....All of the true Masters of the universe are there to greet you.... They embrace you....They honor you... Allow yourself to receive it and feel it all the way down to the core of your being.... The Grand Master comes up to you and says, "Hello, welcome. I'm so proud of you for what you have done to get here."....And it asks you, "Do you have the keys for healing?" ....And you say, "Yes, I have the keys for healing."....And it asks you, "Will you remember them?"....And you say, "Yes, I will remember them.".... And it asks you, "Will you make sure they are not lost?"....And you say, "Yes, I will make sure that they are not lost."....And it asks you, "Are you a Reiki Master?".... And you say, "Yes, I am a Reiki Master."....And it asks you, "What will you do with these keys to healing that you have found?".

Now the Grand Master gives you a gift.... This energy gift is meant to be placed within your body when you get back to it, and it will remind you all the way down to the cellular level that you are a Reiki Master and to honor yourself for that. It tells you where to put it in your physical form when you get back and how to activate it.....It's time to go now....The Grand Master honors you again,....embracing you.....congratulating you again for the step you have taken into mastery. The other masters once again honor you..... It's time to go now, but you know that you can come back here anytime to join with them.....They are always with you on a spirit level....Now, walk back through the doorway, and your Reiki Master is there congratulating you and telling you how it feels about you completing your journey into mastery.

And now your ladder has turned into a fireman's pole, and you're going to slide all the way down the fireman's pole, all the way down into your body....So here you are, halfway between the moon and the earth....A mile above the city....On the roof of this building....Down through the ceiling of this room....Orchestrating yourself so that you go right down into your body....All the way down to your toes....And now you're going to take the gift the Grand Master gave you and place it within you, where he told you to....Now, you're going to take three deep breaths. As you breathe in, you're going to breathe in that quantum leap in consciousness that you've taken. As you breathe out, you're going to reprogram every cell to be a Reiki Master.

So, breathing in....quantum leap in consciousness....

Breathing out....programming every cell to be a Reiki Master.

Breathing in....quantum leap in consciousness...

Breathing out....programming every cell to be a Reiki Master, one more time, Breathing in....quantum leap in consciousness.

Breathing out....programming every cell to be a Reiki Master.

I'm going to count from one to three, and when I get to three, you will be wide awake, fully alert, and feeling wonderful, knowing that every cell of your body has been attuned to Master Degree Reiki.

One, every cell all the way down to the DNA is attuned to Master Degree Reiki.... Two, it's a matter of allowing yourself to know that and to honor that....

Three, awake, feeling wonderful, stretching your arms and legs, wiggling your toes, feeling terrific!

Have each student talk about their experience *(who they met as their Reiki Master)*.

Understanding Auras

Essential Knowledge for Reiki Level 3 Students

More is taught on this subject matter in my book,
"Secrets of a Healer – Magic of Reiki (Vol X)

Trade paperback ISBN: 978-1-7772220-0-0
eBook ISBN 978-1-7772220-1-7

Introduction to Auras

An aura is an electromagnetic energy field that surrounds and permeates the physical body. This field reflects our physical, emotional, mental, and spiritual states. Understanding auras is crucial in Reiki as they play a significant role in the healing process.

What is an Aura?

1. Energy Field: The aura is composed of layers of energy that extend beyond the physical body. Each layer corresponds to different aspects of our being.
2. Colors and Patterns: Auras can display various colors and patterns, each representing different emotional, mental, and spiritual states. These colors can change based on a person's mood, health, and spiritual condition.

Importance of Auras in Reiki

1. Diagnosis and Healing: Reiki practitioners can diagnose imbalances and blockages in a person's energy field by understanding and perceiving auras. This ability allows for more precise and effective healing sessions.
2. Chakra Connection: Auras are closely linked to the chakras, the energy centers in the body. An imbalance in the aura often indicates an issue with one or more chakras.
3. Energy Flow: The aura reflects the flow of life force energy (Reiki) in and around the body. A healthy aura signifies a balanced and harmonious flow of energy.

Why Level 3 Students Need to Understand Auras

1. Advanced Healing Techniques:
   - Aura Cleansing: At the Master Level, students learn advanced techniques for cleansing and balancing the aura. This process involves removing negative energies and enhancing the flow of positive energy.
   - Chakra Balancing: Understanding the aura allows Masters to perform more effective chakra balancing, ensuring that each energy center is functioning optimally.
2. Enhanced Perception:
   - Intuitive Abilities: Master Level students often develop heightened intuitive abilities, allowing them to perceive and interpret the aura's colors and patterns more accurately.

- Energy Sensitivity: Greater sensitivity to energy fields enables Masters to detect subtle imbalances and address them before they manifest physically or emotionally.

3. Teaching and Attuning Others:
    - Student Guidance: When teaching Reiki, Masters must guide students in developing their ability to perceive and understand auras. This knowledge helps new practitioners become more effective healers.
    - Attunement Process: During attunements, understanding the aura is crucial. Masters need to ensure that the student's aura is clear and receptive to the Reiki energy being transmitted.

Practical Applications in Level 3 Training

4. Aura Reading Practice:
    - Exercises and Techniques: Masters teach students exercises to practice seeing and feeling auras. This practice enhances their ability to work with energy fields.
    - Interpretation Skills: Students learn to interpret the colors and patterns they perceive, providing valuable insights into the client's well-being.

5. Aura Cleansing Methods:
    - Hands-on Techniques: Students practice hands-on techniques for cleansing the aura, such as sweeping motions, Reiki symbols, and visualizations.
    - Tools and Aids: Masters may introduce tools like crystals, sage, or sound therapy to aid in aura cleansing.

6. Integration with Reiki Symbols:

- Symbol Usage: Students learn to integrate Reiki symbols, such as the Cho Ku Rei (Power Symbol) and the Dai Ko Myo (Master Symbol), into their aura healing practices.
- Enhanced Energy Flow: Using symbols in aura work enhances the flow of Reiki energy, promoting deeper and more comprehensive healing.

Understanding and working with auras is a fundamental aspect of Reiki Level 3 training. It equips students with the knowledge and skills needed for advanced healing, enhances their intuitive abilities, and prepares them to teach and attune others effectively. Reiki practitioners can provide more holistic and powerful healing sessions by mastering aura techniques, contributing to their growth as Reiki Masters.

Advanced Reiki Practices for Level 3 Students

Types of Reiki Session Choices:

1. Physical Healing
2. Distant Healing
   - d) Visualization
   - e) Full Body Absentee Treatment Hand
   - f) Sandwich Treatment
3. Mental Healing
4. Emotional Healing
5. Spiritual Healing
   - a. Chakra Clearing
   - b. Harmonizing Chakras
   - c. Grounding Exercise
   - d. Casual Plane Work

Deepen your understanding and mastery of Reiki by focusing on techniques such as clearing, harmonizing chakras, grounding exercises, and causal plane work. These practices will enhance your healing abilities and spiritual connections.

Chakra Clearing

Understanding Chakras:

- Seven Main Energy Centers: Chakras are the seven main energy centers in your body, each associated with specific types of energy. These include:
  1. Root Chakra (Muladhara): Associated with survival, grounding, and material needs.
  2. Sacral Chakra (Svadhisthana): Linked to creativity, sexuality, and emotions.
  3. Solar Plexus Chakra (Manipura): Connected with willpower, personal power, and emotions.
  4. Heart Chakra (Anahata): Represents unconditional love, compassion, and healing.
  5. Throat Chakra (Vishuddha): Governs communication, expression, and truth.
  6. Third Eye Chakra (Ajna): Associated with intuition, insight, and self-mastery.
  7. Crown Chakra (Sahasrara): Related to spiritual connection and enlightenment.

Why Clear Chakras:

1. Energy Flow: Clear chakras ensure the free flow of Reiki energy, enhancing your ability to heal and connect spiritually. Blockages can lead to physical, mental, emotional, and spiritual disharmony.

How to Clear Chakras:

Meditation Practice: Regularly practice a chakra-clearing meditation to maintain optimal energy flow. To start, aim to do this daily for the best results.

1. **Negative Energy Chakra Clearing Meditation** with Dr. Constance Santego, YouTube
   https://youtu.be/4cYKHYDLUlo

2. **Clear with Chakra Cord Meditation:**

   - Lie down or sit comfortably.
   - Imagine the ***base/root chakra*** on your body. Imagine it is <u>red</u> in color and the shape of a lotus flower (like a lilypad flower).
     - Imagine this <u>red</u> flower opening up and any Aka cords attached being removed *(the Hawaiians believe we have attachments—imaginary cords—to people. Remove by imagining they are being wiped away, like removing a telephone cord).*
     - We do not cut the cords; we remove them like roots forever.
     - Once all the cords are removed, seal the flower with a clear bubble.
   - Move up to the ***sacral/hara/spleen chakra*** on your body. Imagine it is <u>orange</u> in color and in the shape of a lotus flower, and any attached Aka cords are removed and then sealed with a clear bubble.
   - Repeat sequence -***Solar plexus chakra***, color is a <u>yellow</u> flower in the shape of a lotus flower, and

any attached Aka cords are removed and then sealed with a clear bubble.

- *Heart chakra,* color is a <u>green</u> flower in the shape of a lotus flower, and any Aka cords attached are removed and then sealed with a clear bubble.
- *Throat chakra* is a <u>blue</u> flower in the shape of a lotus flower, and any attached Aka cords are removed and then sealed with a clear bubble.
- **Brow/third eye chakra**, color is an <u>indigo</u> flower in the shape of a lotus flower, and any Aka cords attached are removed and then sealed with a clear bubble.
- **Crown chakra,** color is a <u>violet</u> flower and in the shape of a lotus flower, and any Aka cords attached are removed then sealed with a clear bubble.

Once completed, imagine a beautiful white light—celestial energy coming

a. down through your head,
b. down your back,
c. then turning up through the root chakra
d. all the way up your spine through all the chakras to the crown chakra. Cleansing all the chakras, forming a rainbow by coming out each chakra, coming out the crown chakra
e. making a fountain of beautiful energy that cleanses your aura.
f. Imagine your feet are connected to the earth and the earth's energy *(a wonderful brown color)* coming up through your body, mixing with the celestial energy, grounding you.

g. Now think of positive affirmations *(e.g. I am confident, I am happy, I am successful, etc.)* And seal the affirmations into your DNA.

h. Lastly, when you are completed, take a breath and, wiggle your fingers and toes, open your eyes…feeling rejuvenated.

3. Clear with Colored Light Meditation:

1. Sense where there is negative energy in your body. If there is more than one area, do this for each.
    a. What color is it?
2. Imagine a part of your body that the color energy will come out of into a cosmic garbage can or be vacuumed out.
3. Imagine crystal clear, sparkly love light energy entering your crown chakra and moving the color out through your body and into the cosmic garbage can.
4. Once the color is all gone and only the clear, sparkly love light energy remains, imagine bring in your favorite color (and make it sparkle).
5. Once this new color has replaced the original clear, sparkly love light energy color, have some flow out into the cosmic garbage can for a moment also, making sure all clear has been removed.
6. When that is complete, ask if any other negative energy areas need to be cleared.
7. If 'yes,' repeat the steps; if 'no,' bring any positive words or affirmations into your body.
8. When completed, take a breath and wiggle your toes, saying, "Feeling wonderful."

Harmonizing Chakras

Importance of Harmonizing:

Balanced Energy: Harmonizing chakras balances energy flow, preventing excess or deficiency in any energy center, which can cause various forms of disharmony.

Techniques for Harmonizing:

1. **Balancing Method 1:**
   - *Hand Placement:* Place one hand on your
     - Root Chakra and the other on your Third Eye Chakra.
   - *Energy Equalization:* Hold until you feel the same energy and temperature at both chakras.
   - *Progression:* Move to the
     - Throat Chakra and Sacral Chakra,
     - then the Heart Chakra and Solar Plexus Chakra, repeating the process.
2. **Balancing Method 2:**
   - Root Chakra Focus: Place one hand on the Root Chakra *(one hand always stays here)* and balance each chakra in sequence.
3. **Balancing Method 3:**
   - Third Eye Focus: Place one hand on the Third Eye Chakra *(one hand always stays here)* and balance each chakra in sequence.

Grounding Exercise

Importance of Grounding:

Connection to Earth: Grounding connects you to the Earth's energy, helping to alleviate excessive thoughts, fears, and worries. It brings stability and balance to your energy field.

Steps for Grounding:

1. Preparation:
   - Relaxed Stance: Stand with your feet shoulder-width apart and close your eyes.
2. Breathing:
   - Deep Breathing: Inhale deeply, releasing all tension as you exhale.
   - Repeat two or three times.
3. Energy Visualization:
   - Left Foot Inhalation: As you breathe in, visualize drawing energy up from the earth through your left foot, up your leg, and into your Root Chakra.
   - Right Foot Exhalation: As you breathe out, visualize the energy flowing down your right leg and back into the earth.
4. Duration: Continue this process for 5 to 10 minutes.

Causal Plane Work

Understanding Reiki Causal Plane Work

Welcome to the advanced teachings of Reiki! In Reiki Level 3 (Shinpiden), you will learn about causal plane work, a powerful technique for connecting with others on a deeper, spiritual level. This method can be particularly useful for building spiritual connections, enhancing your practice, and even attracting like-minded individuals or clients.

What is the Causal Plane?

The causal plane is a higher level of consciousness where our souls can interact and communicate beyond the physical and mental planes. It is often referred to as the "soul level" or "dream state," and it is here that we can connect with others on a profound spiritual level. This work is done while you are in a meditative or semi-conscious state, such as just before sleep.

Why is Causal Plane Work Important in Reiki?

Causal plane work allows you to:

- **Build Spiritual Connections**: Connect with the higher selves of others, including potential clients, students, or partners.
- **Enhance Healing**: Send healing intentions to those in need, regardless of physical distance.
- **Manifest Goals**: Attract individuals and opportunities that align with your spiritual and professional goals.

How to Perform Reiki Causal Plane Work

Here is a step-by-step guide to performing causal plane work:

1. Preparation:
    - **Create a Calm Environment:** Find a quiet space where you won't be disturbed. Make sure the environment is comfortable and conducive to meditation.
    - **Relax:** Begin by relaxing your body and mind. Take a few deep breaths to center yourself.
2. Entering the Meditative State:
    - **Half-Asleep State:** This work is best done right before you fall a sleep when you are in a half-awake, half-asleep state. This state of consciousness is optimal for accessing the causal plane.
    - **Set Your Intention:** Clearly state your intention for the causal plane work. For example, you might want to connect with potential clients or send healing energy to someone in need.
3. Affirmation:
    - **Repeat the Affirmation:** As you relax and prepare to enter sleep, repeat the following affirmation: "Tonight, on the causal (or dream, or astral) plane, I am going to send out my Being (or soul, or spirit) to find all of the Beings whose bodies, minds, spirits, and emotions can benefit from the Reiki skills and services I have to offer and from whose interaction I will benefit emotionally and spiritually."

- **Repetition:** If you wake up in the middle of the night, repeat the affirmation to reinforce your intention.

4. Extended Affirmation (Optional):
   - **Further Connection:** For the next three nights, add an extension to your affirmation: "I would like to ask their higher Being to communicate with them as to exactly where to find me."

5. Visualize the Connection:
   - **Imagining the Meeting:** As you drift off to sleep, visualize your soul or spirit reaching out and connecting with others on the causal plane. Picture this interaction as clearly as possible, focusing on the positive exchange of energy and intentions.

6. Upon Waking:
   - **Reflect and Journal:** When you wake up, take a few moments to reflect on any dreams or impressions you had during the night. Write these down in a journal, as they may contain insights or messages from the causal plane.

7. Benefits of Causal Plane Work
   - **Enhanced Spiritual Awareness:**
     - Deepen your connection with your higher self and others on a spiritual level.
     - Attracting Clients and Opportunities:
     - By setting the intention to connect with those who can benefit from your Reiki practice, you may attract new clients or opportunities aligned with your goals.
   - **Sending Healing Energy:**

- Extend your healing reach by sending Reiki energy to individuals, even when they are not physically present.
- **Building a Spiritual Network:**
  - Strengthen your spiritual network by connecting with like-minded individuals who share your values and vision.

Practical Tips

- Consistency:
  - Practice causal plane work regularly to strengthen your ability to connect and communicate on this level.
- Open Mind:
  - Keep an open mind and be receptive to the messages and connections you receive. They may come in unexpected forms.
- Self-Care:
  - Ensure you are well-rested and take care of your physical and emotional well-being, as this enhances your ability to perform causal plane work effectively.

Incorporating causal plane work into your Reiki practice will expand your ability to connect, heal, and grow spiritually. This advanced technique opens up new dimensions of interaction and manifestation, enriching your personal and professional Reiki journey.

Reiki Master = Teacher

Teaching Reiki Level 3: Master Level and the Ability to Teach and Initiate

Reiki Level 3, also known as the Master Level, is a significant milestone in a Reiki practitioner's journey. This level enhances the practitioner's healing abilities and empowers them with the knowledge and skills needed to teach Reiki and initiate others through attunements. Here is an overview of what it means to reach the Master Level in Reiki and its responsibilities.

Master Level Overview

1. Master Symbols
    *   The Master Level introduces the Raku, Dai Ko Myo, and the White Light symbols.
2. Advanced Techniques
    *   Reiki Masters learn advanced healing techniques, such as aura clearing, chakra balancing, and spiritual healing practices.
    *   These techniques allow Masters to provide comprehensive and profound healing sessions.
3. Spiritual Growth
    *   The Master Level focuses on the practitioner's spiritual development, encouraging them to deepen their connection with the universal life force energy and their higher self.

- This level promotes personal empowerment, self-awareness, and enlightenment.
- Ability to Teach and Initiate

4. Teaching Reiki
    - Curriculum Development: Reiki Masters are trained to develop and organize a curriculum for teaching Reiki Levels 1, 2, and 3. This includes creating lesson plans, instructional materials, and practical exercises.
    - Class Management: Masters learn how to manage a class effectively, ensuring each student receives the attention and guidance they need.

5. Conducting Attunements
    - Attunement Process: Masters are taught the detailed process of performing Reiki attunements. This includes the sacred rituals and symbols used in all levels, from Reiki Level 1 (Shoden) to Reiki Level 3 (Shinpiden), each with its specific attunement process and requirements.
    - Detailed Responsibilities of a Reiki Master

6. Performing Attunements
    - Level 1 Attunement: This attunement opens the student's energy channels to allow them to connect with Reiki energy. The process involves using the Cho Ku Rei (Power Symbol) to empower and protect the student.
    - Level 2 Attunement: This includes the introduction of the Sei He Ki (Emotional Healing Symbol) and Hon Sha Ze Sho Nen (Distant Healing Symbol), further enhancing the student's healing capabilities.

- Level 3 Attunement: The Master Level attunement involves the Dai Ko Myo (Master Symbol) and is a profound spiritual initiation that enables the student to teach and perform attunements.

7. Teaching Methodology
   - Instruction: Masters are responsible for teaching the theoretical aspects of Reiki, including its history, principles, and ethical guidelines.
   - Practical Application: They guide students through hands-on practice sessions, demonstrating and supervising Reiki techniques and hand positions.
   - Mentorship: Providing ongoing support and mentorship to students is a key responsibility. Masters help students integrate Reiki into their daily lives and practice.

8. Ethical Considerations
   - Integrity: Reiki Masters must adhere to high ethical standards, maintaining the integrity and purity of the Reiki teachings.
   - Respect for Students: They must respect each student's spiritual path and provide a safe, supportive learning environment.
   - Confidentiality: Ensuring confidentiality and trust between the practitioner and students is paramount.

9. Personal and Professional Development
   - Continuous Learning: Masters should commit to ongoing personal and professional development, staying updated with the latest Reiki practices and insights.

- Community Engagement: Engaging with the Reiki community through workshops, Reiki circles, and other events helps foster a sense of belonging and continuous learning.

10. Creating a Healing Environment
   - Sacred Space: Masters should create a serene and energetically clear space for teaching and healing. This environment supports the attunement process and enhances the learning experience.
   - Preparation: Properly preparing the space and themselves energetically before each class or session ensures the best possible outcomes.

11. Developing Instructional Materials
   - Manuals and Handouts: Providing comprehensive manuals and handouts helps students retain and reference the material.
   - Visual Aids: Visual aids like charts and diagrams can enhance understanding, especially for visual learners.

The Role of a Reiki Master

1. Healer
   - As a healer, the Reiki Master continues to provide advanced healing sessions to clients, addressing deeper levels of healing and promoting overall well-being.

2. Teacher
   - As a teacher, the Master shares knowledge and techniques with students, empowering them to become effective Reiki practitioners.

3. Initiator
   - As an initiator, the Master conducts attunements, facilitating the transmission of Reiki energy to new practitioners and enabling them to heal themselves and others.
4. Guide and Mentor
   - The Master acts as a guide and mentor, supporting students on their Reiki journey, offering advice, and helping them navigate challenges and spiritual growth.

Reiki Level 3, the Master Level, is a transformative stage in a Reiki practitioner's journey. It not only enhances their healing abilities but also bestows the sacred responsibility of teaching and initiating others into the practice of Reiki. By embracing the roles of healer, teacher, initiator, and mentor, a Reiki Master contributes to spreading Reiki's healing and spiritual benefits, fostering a community of enlightened and empowered individuals. This profound journey requires dedication, continuous learning, and a commitment to maintaining the integrity and purity of the Reiki tradition.

Preparing to Teach Reiki

1. Personal Preparation
   - Master Level Certification: Ensure you have completed your own Reiki Master training and have sufficient experience with Reiki practice.
   - Continuous Practice: Maintain a regular Reiki practice for personal growth and energy maintenance.
   - Lesson Planning: Develop detailed lesson plans for each level, including objectives, activities, and materials needed.
2. Setting Up Your Classes
   - Location: Choose a quiet, comfortable, and energetically clear space for teaching.
   - Materials: Prepare necessary materials such as handouts, manuals, charts, and any required tools for attunements.
   - Class Size: Decide on the class size that allows for personal attention and effective teaching.

Teaching Reiki Level 1: The Foundation

Objective: Introduce students to the basics of Reiki, including its history, principles, and basic techniques. By the end of this level, students should be able to perform self-healing and provide healing to others.

1. Introduction to Reiki
   - History: Teach the history and origin of Reiki, including Dr. Mikao Usui's contributions.
   - Principles: Explain the five Reiki principles and their importance in daily life.
2. Energy and Chakras
   - Understanding Energy: Discuss the concept of life force energy and its significance in Reiki.
   - Chakras: Introduce the chakra system and its relevance to energy healing.
3. Attunement
   - Attunement Process: Conduct the Level 1 attunement ceremony, opening the students' energy channels to Reiki energy.
   - Experience Sharing: Allow students to share their experiences and feelings after the attunement.
4. Reiki Symbols
   - Introduction to Symbols: Introduce the Reiki symbol – Cho Ku Rei (Power Symbol).
5. Hand Positions
   - Self-Healing: Demonstrate and practice the hand positions for self-healing.

6. Practice Sessions
    - Guided Practice: Lead guided practice sessions for self-healing.
    - Feedback: Provide feedback and answer questions to help students refine their technique.
7. Homework and Daily Practice
    - Daily Reiki Practice: Encourage students to practice self-Reiki daily.
    - Journaling: Suggest keeping a Reiki journal to document their experiences and progress.

Teaching Reiki Level 2: Deepening the Connection

Objective: Introduce students to Reiki symbols and advanced mental, emotional, and distant healing techniques. By the end of this level, students should be able to use Reiki symbols effectively and conduct distant healing sessions.

1. Review of Level 1
   - Revisit Fundamentals: Briefly review the concepts and techniques learned in Level 1.
2. Attunement
   - Level 2 Attunement: Conduct the Level 2 attunement ceremony, empowering students to use the symbols.
   - Experience Sharing: Allow students to share their experiences and insights after the attunement.
3. Reiki Symbols
   - Introduction to Symbols: Introduce the two Reiki symbols –Sei He Ki (Emotional Healing Symbol), and Hon Sha Ze Sho Nen (Distant Healing Symbol).
   - Drawing and Usage: Teach how to draw each symbol and explain its specific uses and benefits.
4. Mental and Emotional Healing
   - Sei He Ki: Demonstrate and practice using the Sei He Ki symbol for mental and emotional healing.
   - Techniques: Teach techniques for addressing specific mental and emotional issues.

5. Hand Positions
   - Healing Others: Teach the hand positions for giving Reiki to others.
6. Distant Healing
   - Hon Sha Ze Sho Nen: Demonstrate and practice using the Hon Sha Ze Sho Nen symbol for distant healing.
   - Methods: Teach different methods for sending distant Reiki, such as visualization and using a proxy.
7. Practice Sessions
   - Advanced Practice: Lead practice sessions using the symbols for self-healing, healing others, and distant healing.
   - Case Studies: Encourage students to share case studies and experiences to enhance learning.
8. Homework and Daily Practice
   - Symbol Practice: Encourage the daily practice of drawing and using symbols.
   - Distant Healing Practice: Suggest regular practice of distant healing sessions.

Teaching Reiki Level 3: Master Level

Objective: Prepare students to become Reiki Masters, enabling them to teach and attune others. This level focuses on mastery of Reiki energy and spiritual growth.

1. Review of Levels 1 and 2
   - Comprehensive Review: Review all concepts, techniques, and symbols learned in Levels 1 and 2.
2. Master Attunement
   - Master Attunement Ceremony: Conduct the Master Level attunement, empowering students with the Master Symbol and the ability to attune others.
   - Experience Sharing: Encourage students to share their experiences and feelings after the attunement.
3. Master Symbol
   - Introduce the Raku, Dai Ko Myo, and White Light symbols, explaining their significance and uses.
   - Drawing and Usage: Teach how to draw and incorporate symbols into Reiki practice.
4. Advanced Techniques
   - Healing Techniques: Teach advanced healing techniques, including aura clearing and chakra balancing.
   - Spiritual Healing: Discuss the role of Reiki in spiritual growth and development.

5. Teaching and Attunements
    - Teaching Methods: Provide guidance on how to teach Reiki to others, including creating lesson plans and managing a class.
    - Attunement Process: Teach the detailed process of performing Reiki attunements for each level.
    - Practical Experience: Allow students to practice giving attunements under supervision.
6. Practice Sessions
    - Master Level Practice: Lead advanced practice sessions focusing on the use of the Master Symbol and advanced techniques.
    - Teaching Practice: Allow students to practice teaching segments of the class and performing attunements.
7. Ongoing Support and Mentoring
    - Continued Guidance: Offer ongoing support and mentoring for new Reiki Masters as they begin to teach and attune others.
8. Community Building: Encourage participation in Reiki circles and communities for continued growth and support.

Teaching Reiki Levels 1-3 involves guiding students through a structured progression of learning and practice. Each level builds upon the previous one, deepening their understanding and connection to Reiki energy. As a Reiki Master Teacher, your role is to provide comprehensive instruction, support, and empowerment to your students, helping them to become confident and effective Reiki practitioners and teachers.

Teaching Guidelines for Reiki Level 3 Students

As a Reiki Level 3 student (Shinpiden), you are now ready to teach and attune others. Here are the essential guidelines for organizing and conducting your Reiki classes.

Advertising Your Classes

1. Details to Include:
    - Place: Clearly state the location of your classes.
    - Date and Time: Specify the dates and times for each class.
    - Offering: Describe what you offer in the class (e.g., Reiki Level 1, 2, or Master).
    - Contact Information: Include your name and phone number for inquiries and registrations.
2. Price: Mention the cost of the class.
    - Typical Time Frame and Pricing:
    - Reiki Level 1 (Shoden):
        1. Duration: 3-4 classes, each 3 hours long.
        2. Price: $150.00
    - Reiki Level 2 (Okuden):
        1. Duration: 3-4 classes, each 3 hours long.
        2. Price: $200.00 - $250.00
    - Reiki Level 3 (Shinpiden) / Master Level:
        1. Duration: 3-4 classes, each 3 hours long.

2. Price: $500.00-$1000.00

Preparing Materials

1. Manuals:
    - Photocopy or Print Manuals: Prepare manuals for your students. You can choose to photocopy existing materials or print new ones.
        - Format Options:
        - Book: Bound manuals.
        - Paper: Loose-leaf format for easy addition of notes.
        - Print: Professionally printed materials for a polished look.
2. Refreshments:
    - Lemon Juice: For the attunement.
    - Water: Provide refreshments for your students to keep them hydrated and energized during class.
    - Cups: Ensure you have enough cups for all participants.

Conducting Your Classes

1. Setting Up:
    - Create a Sacred Space: Ensure the teaching area is calm, clean, and energetically clear. Use candles, incense, or calming music to enhance the atmosphere.

- Seating Arrangement: Arrange seating to facilitate interaction and visibility for all participants.
2. Class Structure:
   - Introduction: Begin each class with an introduction outlining the goals and agenda for the session.
   - Teaching and Demonstration: Explain the concepts, demonstrate techniques, and encourage hands-on practice.
   - Q&A Sessions: Allow time for questions and answers to clarify any doubts.
   - Practice: Provide ample time for students to practice the techniques on themselves and others.
3. Attunements:
   - Perform Attunements: Conduct attunements for each level as part of the class, ensuring each student is properly attuned to the Reiki energy.
   - Experience Sharing: Encourage students to share their experiences and feelings after the attunement.
4. Closing:
   - Review and Reflect: Summarize the key points of the class and provide feedback.
   - Assign Homework: Give students homework or practice assignments to reinforce their learning.
   - Distribute Certificates: Hand out certificates of completion to students who have successfully completed the course.

Additional Tips

1. Clear Communication:
   - Maintain clear and open communication with your students. Provide them with your contact information for any follow-up questions or support.
2. Ongoing Support:
   - Offer ongoing support and mentorship to your students. Encourage them to join Reiki circles or practice groups to continue their growth and learning.
3. Continuous Learning:
   - Stay updated with the latest Reiki practices and techniques. Continuously improve your own skills and knowledge to provide the best teaching experience.

By following these guidelines, you can effectively organize, advertise, and conduct your Reiki classes, ensuring a valuable and enriching experience for your students.

Attunement Procedure for Each Reiki Level

Attunements

1. Introduction to the Course:
   - Introduce the course and outline what the students can expect during the session.
2. Initiate the Attunement:
   - Invocation:
     - Meditate and bring down your own Reiki Master in spirit to assist you during the attunement process.
3. Opening the Chakras:
   - Crown Chakra:
     - Position: Stand behind the student.
     - Action: Open the student's Crown Chakra using the Master Symbol and draw the Raku symbol.
     - Visualization: Imagine the Reiki energy flowing into all areas.
4. Symbols:
   - Crown Chakra
     - Position: Stand behind the student.
     - Action: Open the student's Crown Chakra,
       - Level 1: Draw the Cho Ku Rei symbol.
       - Level 2: Draw the Sei He Ki symbol.
       - Master Level: Draw the Raku symbol.
   - Heart Chakra:

- Position: Move to the front of the student.
- Action: Open the student's Heart Chakra.
- Symbols:
    - Level 1: Draw the Cho Ku Rei symbol.
    - Level 2: Draw the Sei He Ki symbol.
    - Master Level: Draw the Raku symbol.
- Hand Chakras:
    - Position: The front of the student.
    - Action: Open the student's Hand Chakras.
    - Symbols:
        - Level 1: Draw the Cho Ku Rei symbol.
        - Level 2: Draw the Sei He Ki symbol.
        - Master Level: Draw the Raku symbol.

5. Hands Position: Close the student's hands into a prayer position.
    - Breath and Energy Connection:
    - Kidney Breath: Both you and the student take a kidney breath while holding the Hui Yin position.
6. Closing the Chakras:
    - Crown Chakra:
        - Position: Return to standing behind the student.

- Action: Close the student's Crown Chakra using the Master Symbol.
7. Finish the Meditation:
   - Conclude the meditation, ensuring both you and the student are grounded and centered.
8. Water Ritual:
   - Perform a water ritual to cleanse and seal the attunement.
9. Discussion:
   - Talk about what happened during the meditation, allowing the student to share their experiences and insights.

Conclude the Course:

Finish with any remaining course information and address any final questions or student comments.

Following this attunement procedure for each level ensures that the students are properly attuned to Reiki energy, enabling them to channel Reiki for themselves and others effectively.

Reiki Certificates Examples

Issuing student certificates is essential to validate their training and accomplishments in Reiki. Here's a detailed guide on handling Reiki certificates at different levels of training.

Types of Certificates

1. Completion Certificates:
   - Awarded when students have successfully met all the requirements of the course.
   - These certificates allow the students to practice Reiki professionally, charge for their services, and obtain a business license.
   - Seal and Stamp: Consider getting a seal and stamp for your certificates to give them an official and professional look.

Requirements for Completion Certificates

1. Finished Classes:
   - The student must attend and complete all scheduled classes for the respective Reiki level.
2. Tests and Assessments:
   - Written Test: Assessing the student's understanding of Reiki principles, symbols, and techniques.
   - Practical Test: Evaluating the student's ability to perform Reiki sessions and use Reiki symbols correctly.
3. Case Studies and Homework:

- Submission of case studies demonstrating the practical application of Reiki on others.
- Completion of assigned homework to reinforce learning and practice.

Issuing Certificates

1. Preparation:
   - Design: Create a professional-looking certificate with the following elements:
   - Student's name
   - Course level (Level 1, Level 2, Master Level)
   - Date of completion
   - Reiki Master's name and signature
   - Seal and stamp (optional, for added authenticity)
   - Paper Quality: Use high-quality paper to print the certificates for a polished appearance.
2. Distribution:
   - Completion Certificate: Awarded to students who have passed all requirements, allowing them to practice Reiki professionally.

Example Certificate Wording

Completion Certificate:

Level 1

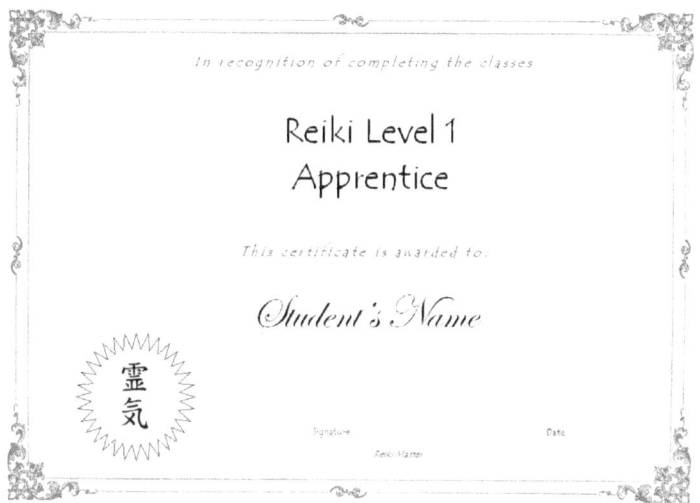

Level 2

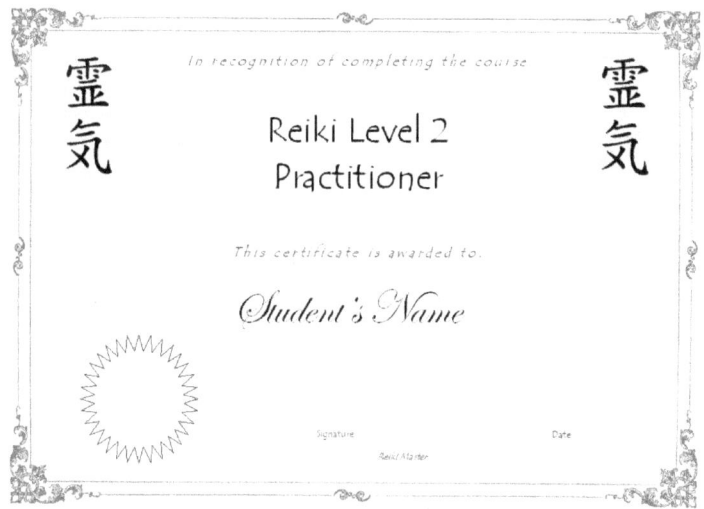

Level 3

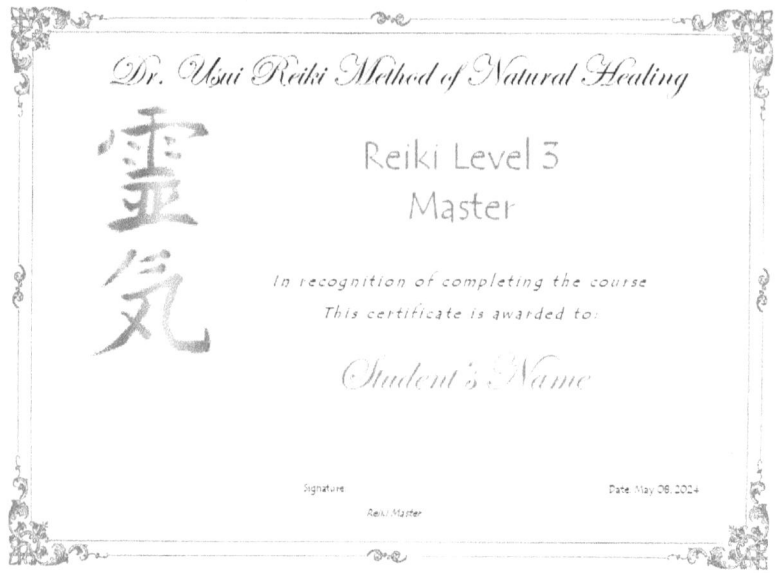

Additional Tips

1. Clear Communication:
   - Clearly explain the difference between completion and participation certificates to your students before the course begins. Ensure they understand the requirements for obtaining a completion certificate.
2. Record Keeping:
   - Maintain accurate records of all issued certificates, including the names of students, dates, and types of certificates awarded. This helps in verifying credentials if needed in the future.

3. Encouragement:
   - Encourage students who receive participation certificates to continue their studies and practice, working towards earning a completion certificate in the future.

Following these guidelines ensures your Reiki certification process is transparent, professional, and meaningful for your students.

Companion Books

More is taught about Energy healing, Chakras, and Reiki in my book,

"Secrets of a Healer – Magic of Reiki (Vol X)

Trade paperback ISBN: 978-1-7772220-0-0

eBook ISBN 978-1-7772220-1-7

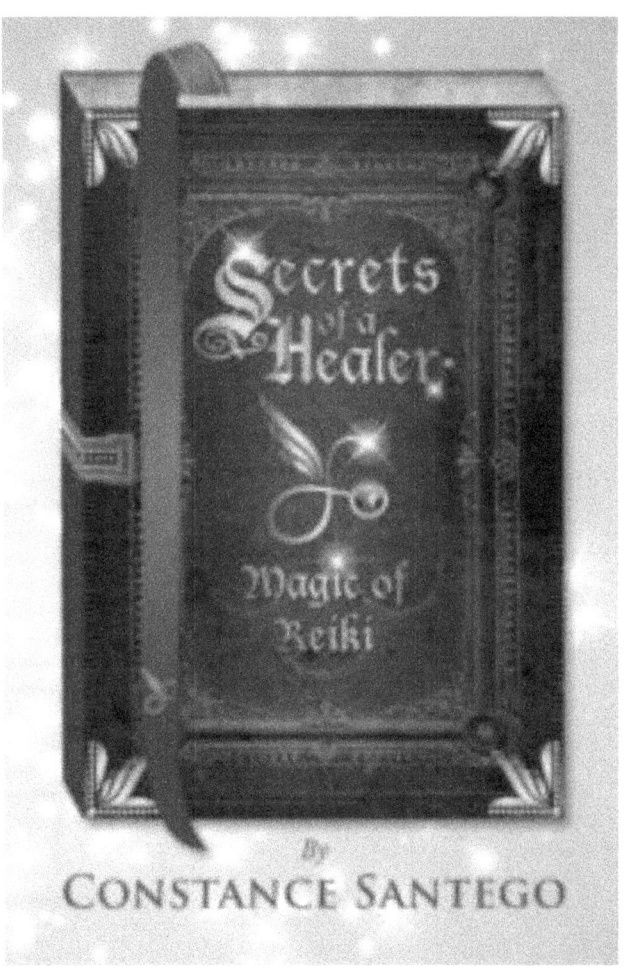

and in my Novel Series,
"The Nine Spiritual Gifts Granted By Spirit"
Vol IV in the series, *"Miracles of a Soul"*

Soft Cover ISBN: 978-1-990062-12-4
eBook ISBN: 978-1-990062-13-1

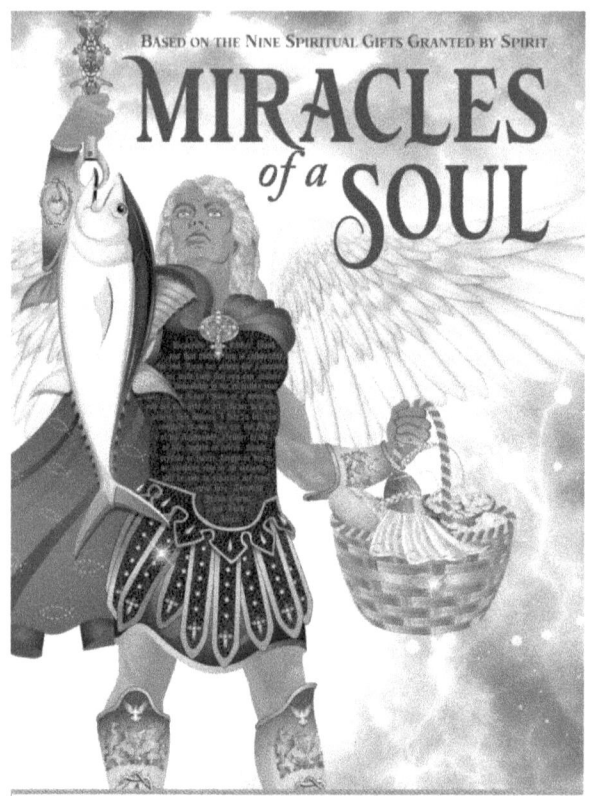

BASED ON THE NINE SPIRITUAL GIFTS GRANTED BY SPIRIT

MIRACLES of a SOUL

A NOVEL
Lexi Constantine's Fifth Adventure
This Time with Archangel Hamied's Help
THE GIFT OF MIRACLES

CONSTANCE SANTEGO

Bibliography

Bibliography

Much of this information was taken from the course information created when I owned the Canadian Institute of Natural Health and Healing Accredited College.

Quantum University www.quantumuniversity.com

Artwork – www.canva.com

Associations - https://iarp.org/history-of-Reiki/

A Suggested Reading List

There are many books available to further your learning on the topics covered in this course; those listed here are some suggestions:

Ascended Masters

King, Godfrey Ray

Unveiled Mysteries (Saint Germain Series; Vol.1).

1989   The Magic Presence (Saint Germain Series; Vol. 2).

Sandweiss, Samuel H.

> 1975   Sai Baba: The Holy Man and the Psychiatrist. San Diego, California: Birth Day Publishing Company

Stone, Joshua David

> 1995   Ascended Masters Light the Way. Sedona, Arizona: Light Technology.   Publications.

Aura and Psychometry

Brennan, Barbara

> 1988   Hands of Light: a Guide to Healing Through the Human Energy Field. Bantam Books.

Chakras

Arguelles, Jose

> 1987   The Mayan Factor: Path Beyond Technology.

Beinfield, Harriet and Korngold, Efrem

> 1991   A Guide to Chinese Medicine. New York: Ballantine Books.

Castaneda, Carlos

> 1974   Tales of Power. New York, New York: Pocket Books

Energy Healing

Brennan, Barbara Ann

> 1987   Hands of Light. New York, New York: Bantam Books.

Guides

Altea, Rosemary

> 1995   The Eagle and the Rose. New York, New York: Warner Books Inc.

Eadie, Betty J.

> 1992   Embraced By The Light. New York: Bantam Books.

> 1996   The Awakening Heart. New York, New York: Pocket Books.

Guggenheim, Bill

> 1995   Hello From Heaven. New York: Bantam Books.

Van Praagh, James

> 1997   Talking to Heaven. New York, New York: Penguin Group

Healing

Steiger, Brad

> 1971   Kahuna Magic. Westchester, Pennsylvania: Whitford Press.

Gienger, Michael

> 2004   Crystal Power, Crystal Healing. London, U.K.: Blandford

Hay, Louise L.

> 1988   Heal Your Body. Carlsbad, California: Hay House, Incorporated.

Pendulums

Graves, Tom

> 1989   The Elements of Pendulum Dowsing. Shaftesbury, Dorset: Element Books.

Lubek, Walter

> 1998   Pendulum Healing Handbook. Twin Lakes, Wisconsin: Lotus Light Publications.

Religion

> The Bible – several versions available.

Baigent, Michael; Leigh, Richard and Lincoln, Henry

> 2005   Holy Blood, Holy Grail Illustrated Edition: The Secret History of Jesus, the Shocking Legacy of the Grail. Delacorte Press.

Brown, Dan

> 2003   The Da Vinci Code. New York, New York: Doubleday

Gardner, Laurence

> 2002   Blood Line of the Holy Grail: The Hidden Legacy of Jesus Revealed. Fair Winds Press.

Symbols

Chetwynd, Tom

> 1982   Dictionary of Symbols. London, Paladin Books: Harper Collins.

Summer Rains, Mary and Greystone, Alex

1996   Guide to Dream Symbols. Charlottesville, Virginia: Harper Roads Publishing Company.

Reiki

Stein, Diane

1995   Essential Reiki, A Complete Guide To An Ancient Healing Art. Freedom, CA, The Crossing Press Inc.

Barnett, Libby and Chambers, Maggie

1996   Reiki Energy Medicine. Rochester Vermont, Healing Arts Press

Foreword by Rand William Lee

1999   The Original Reiki Handbook of Dr. Mikao Usui. Shangri-La, Lotus Press

Honervogt, Tanmaya

1998   The Power of Reiki. New York, New York, Henry Holt and Company Inc.

General

Becker, Dr. Robert O. and Gary Selden

1985   The Body Electric. New York: Quill, William Morrow.

Cameron, Julia

1992   The Artist's Way. New York, New York: Jeremy P. Tarcher/Putnam.

Davidson, Gustav

> 1967   Dictionary of Angels. New York, New York: The
> Free Press.

Emoto, Masaru

> 2004 The Hidden Messages in Water. Hillsboro, Oregon:
> Beyond Words Publications.

Kroeger, Hanna

> 1973   The Pendulum, The Bible and Your Survival. Hanna
> Kroeger Publications.

Morgan, Marlo

> 1991   Mutant Message Down Under. New York, New
> York: Harper Collins.

Redfield, James

> 1993   The Celestine Prophecy. New York, New York:
> Warner Books Inc.

Walsch, Neale Donald

> 1996   Conversations With God. New York, New York:
> G.P. Putnam & Sons.

Textbook

> Prescription for Nutritional Healing
> ISBN 7-35918-33077-1

Suggested Internet Resources

There are literally millions of sites on the internet. You may do a "search" to get a list of sites that contain your keywords. Only by visiting them will you be able to determine which are helpful to you. Don't forget that from one site, you can often be directed to related sites.

What follows is simply a sample of Internet Resources. You are encouraged to extend your search to topics of interest to you.

Aura

http://www.bioenergyfields.org/index.asp?secid=3&subsecid=0

Chakras

https://www.curativesoul.com/Chakras#.XrBe4qhKgdU

https://www.learning-mind.com/7-Chakras-issues/

https://chopra.com/articles/what-is-a-Chakra

https://Chakrasincense.com/
https://diannetrussell.com/energy/articles-2/truth-about-colour/

World Religions

https://www.history.com/topics/religion/bible

http://www.mnsu.edu/emuseum/cultural/religion/

http://www.religion-cults.com/

http://en.wikipedia.org/wiki/Major_world_religions

- Islam
  http://images.google.ca/images?svnum=10&hl=en&lr=&q=
  islam+symbol&btnG=Search

- Christianity
  http://images.google.ca/images?svnum=10&hl=en&lr=&q=christia
  nity+symbol&btnG=Search

- Hinduism
  http://images.google.ca/images?q=Hinduism+symbol&ndsp=20&s
  vnum=10&hl=en&lr=&start=60&sa=N

  http://www.mnsu.edu/emuseum/cultural/religion/hinduism/belie
  fs.html

- Buddhism
  http://www.mnsu.edu/emuseum/cultural/religion/buddhism/beli
  efs.html

- Judaism
  http://images.google.ca/images?q=judaism+symbols&ndsp=20&sv
  num=10&hl=en&lr=&start=40&sa=N

- Traditional Chinese
  http://images.google.ca/images?q=Tao+symbols&ndsp=20&svnu
  m=10&hl=en&lr=&start=80&sa=N

- Bahai faith
  http://images.google.ca/images?svnum=10&hl=en&lr=&q=bahai+f
  aith+symbol&btnG=Search

https://en.wikipedia.org/wiki/Sanskrit

https://www.ancient.eu/Sanskrit/

Ascended Masters

http://www.dci.dk/en/mtrl/saibabaeng.html

http://www.srisathyasai.org.in/Pages/SriSathyaSaiBaba/Introductio n.htm

http://www.greatdreams.com/masters/ascended-masters.htm

http://en.wikipedia.org/wiki/Ascended_master#Examples_of_asce nded_masters

http://www.theascendedmasters.com/

http://en.wikipedia.org/wiki/Count_of_St_Germain

Kirlian Photography

http://images.google.ca/images?svnum=10&hl=en&lr=&q=kirlian+ photography&btnG=Search

Misc. Info

http://www.zeitgeistmovie.com/Zietgeist

https://www.goodreads.com/book/similar/130686-the-holy-blood-and-the-holy-grail

Tuning Forks

www.Luminati.com
www.somaenergetics.com
https://www.allbodycare.com/tuning-fork-therapy-sound-healing/
https://medium.com/meducated-org/how-to-heal-your-body-by-using-the-frequency-of-life-9307af550fbb

Suggested Video Resources

The film industry has released many movies depicting metaphysical beliefs and phenomena; just a few are listed here. While they are fantasy, they may improve your understanding of topics addressed in this course.

1999   What Dreams May Come   Directed by Vincent Ward

1999   The Sixth Sense   Directed by M. Night Shayamalan

1999   The Matrix   Directed by Andy Wachowski and Larry Wachowski

1999   Ninth Gate   Directed by Roman Polanski

1999   Patch Adams   Directed by Tom Shadyac

1996   Michael   Directed by Nora Ephron

1996   Phenomenon   Directed by John Turtletaub

1991   Stigmata   Directed by Rupert Wainright

1990   Ghost   Directed by Jerry Zucker

Message From The Author

To this day, Reiki still mystifies me. I am in awe every day of the power of this life-force energy. Powerful, yet so gentle!

The old saying, 'Wonders never cease to amaze me,' *meaning an expression of surprise used when something unusual or unexpected happens,* really is appropriate for this modality. You will never tire of the miracles you will witness.

Shift happens… Create magic!
Dr. Constance

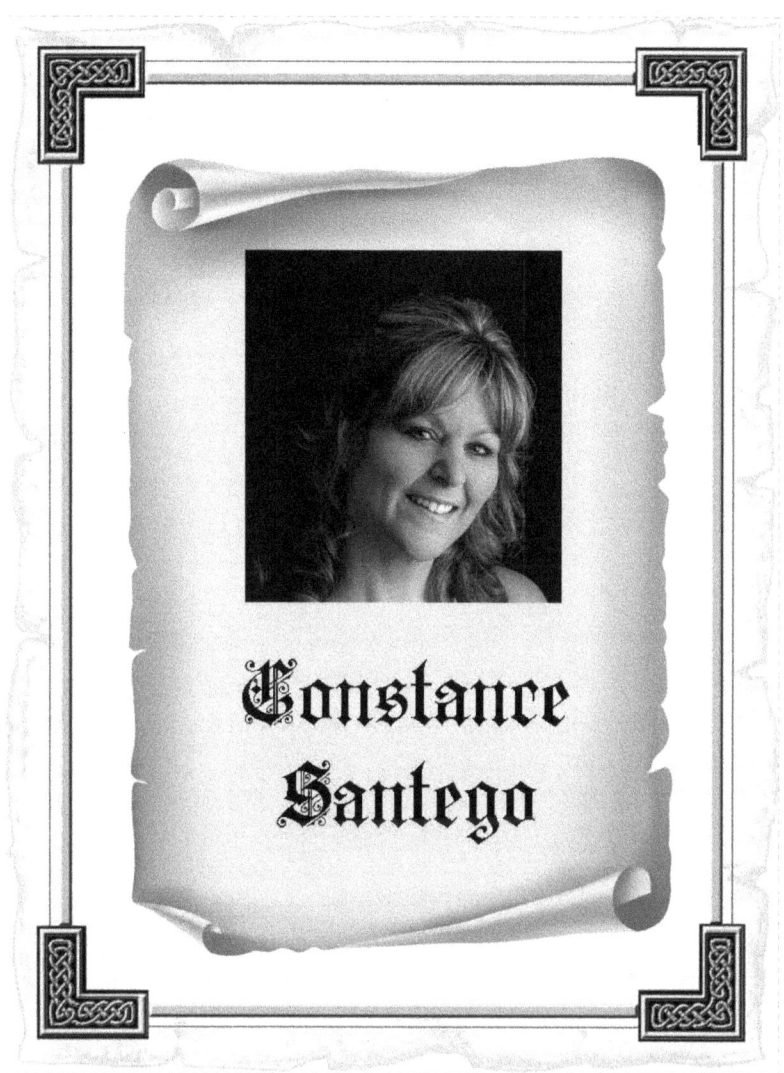

Constance Santego

Dream BIGGER!

Dr. Constance Santego is a highly respected expert in the field of holistic health and spiritual healing. She holds a Grand Reiki Master title and, with over twenty years of experience teaching courses on these subjects, has developed a deep understanding of the interconnectedness of the mind, body, and spirit in achieving overall well-being.

Dr. Santego holds a Ph.D. and Doctorate in Natural Medicine, which has provided her with a comprehensive understanding of alternative healing modalities and their application in promoting optimal health. Her educational background has equipped her with the knowledge to address health concerns holistically, considering the physical, emotional, and spiritual aspects of an individual's well-being.

Throughout her career, Dr. Santego has been committed to sharing her knowledge and empowering others to take control of their health and healing. She uniquely can blend scientific research and traditional wisdom, creating a bridge between conventional and alternative medicine.

In her "Secrets of a Healer" educational series, Dr. Santego draws upon her vast experience and expertise to captivate readers with her insights and teachings. She takes readers on a transformative journey, delving into the realms of holistic health, spirituality, and self-discovery. Through her writing, she aims to inspire individuals to tap into their own innate healing abilities and embrace a balanced and harmonious approach to well-being.

Dr. Santego's work has touched the lives of many, guiding them toward a more profound understanding of themselves and their connection to the world around them. Her series is a beacon of wisdom, offering practical tools and techniques for personal growth and transformation.

Overall, Dr. Constance Santego's blend of knowledge, experience, and passion makes her a captivating figure in holistic health and spiritual healing. Her contributions through teaching, writing, and her spellbinding series continue to inspire and empower individuals on their journeys toward well-being and self-discovery.

ALSO AVAILABLE

Play the game *Ikona* – Discover Your Inner Genie

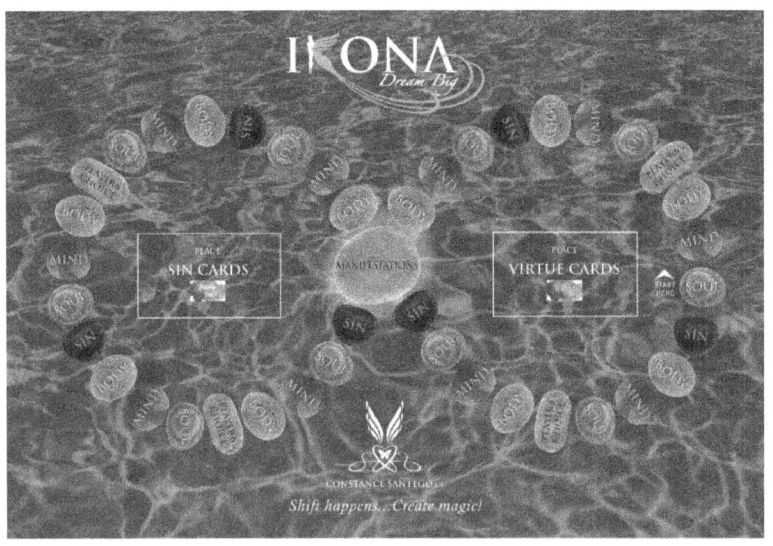

For additional information on

Constance Santego's

wide range of Motivational Products, Coaching Sessions,
Spiritual Retreats,
Live Events and Educational Programs

Go to

www.ConstanceSantego.ca

Follow on Instagram - Constance_Santego and
Facebook - constancesantegoo

Subscribe and receive Free Information and Meditations on
my
YouTube Channel - Constance Santego

www.ingramcontent.com/pod-product-compliance
Lightning Source LLC
Chambersburg PA
CBHW051142120626
46547CB00012B/919